KU-266-101

Robert A. Norman (Ed.)

Common Treatments in Preventive Dermatology

How to Treat Your Patient

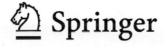

Springer

Editor
Dr. Robert A. Norman
Nova Southeastern University
Ft. Lauderdale, FL, USA and
Private Practice
Tampa
FL, USA

ALISTAIR MACKENZIE LIBRARY
Barcode: 3690289151
Class no: WR 100 NOR

ISBN 978-0-85729-852-2   e-ISBN 978-0-85729-853-9
DOI 10.1007/978-0-85729-853-9
Springer London Dordrecht Heidelberg New York

British Library Cataloguing in Publication Data
A catalogue record for this book is available from the British Library

Library of Congress Control Number: 2011933835

© Springer-Verlag London Limited 2012
Apart from any fair dealing for the purposes of research or private study, or criticism or review, as permitted under the Copyright, Designs and Patents Act 1988, this publication may only be reproduced, stored or transmitted, in any form or by any means, with the prior permission in writing of the publishers, or in the case of reprographic reproduction in accordance with the terms of licenses issued by the Copyright Licensing Agency. Enquiries concerning reproduction outside those terms should be sent to the publishers.
The use of registered names, trademarks, etc., in this publication does not imply, even in the absence of a specific statement, that such names are exempt from the relevant laws and regulations and therefore free for general use.
Product liability: The publisher can give no guarantee for information about drug dosage and application thereof contained in this book. In every individual case the respective user must check its accuracy by consulting other pharmaceutical literature.

Printed on acid-free paper

Springer is part of Springer Science+Business Media (www.springer.com)

(LINAGHIL AGUSAGHAGUL ...)

Foreword

In his latest books, Dr. Rob Norman introduces us to the intriguing concept of preventive dermatology. While dermatologists have long been patient advocates and have stressed vigorously the importance of sun avoidance and protection, there is still much more that we can do to prevent disease.

Dr. Norman and his skilled coterie of collaborators discuss two distinct types of prevention in dermatology: the prevention of skin diseases and the prevention of systemic disorders, some with only very indirect connections to the skin. The first is fairly well known to dermatologists; the second is truly an emerging concept of great importance.

Educational efforts to prevent or at least control skin disease may range from the proper use of sunscreens to weight loss in psoriatic patients, the avoidance of trigger factors in rosacea, proper skin care in atopic dermatitis, or adoption of a low-fat diet to decrease the incidence of actinic keratosis and non-melanoma skin cancer. Another good example, is the use of vaccines to protect against diseases such as herpes zoster and genital HPV infection in females.

This book, however, looks beyond the prevention of skin diseases to suggest that dermatologists view their patients through a more holistic lens. This means treating the entire patient not just the skin. Thus Dr. Norman suggests that we be more proactive in addressing health issues such as obesity, smoking, stress management, and nutrition. Consider, for example, the psoriatic patient, whose disease must now be treated as a systemic disorder predisposing to the very serious risks of the metabolic triad.

As dermatologists, we deal with numerous chronic diseases, seeing some patients repeatedly over many years. This longitudinal interaction offers an excellent platform for the practice of preventive dermatology.

Read and enjoy this book. It could make you a better dermatologist.

Professor and Chairman   John E. Wolf Jr., M.D.
Department of Dermatology

Preface

It seems almost counter-intuitive to cover dermatology prevention, because so much of what we do in dermatology is based on repair and restructuring of skin maladies. But with the shortage of dermatology providers and the shift to cosmetics and procedures, it is urgent to make sure our patients are given a fair chance to succeed in the fast-changing world of modern healthcare. Although we are specialists in the care of the skin, we are health care providers first, and should treat our patients with a holistic and caring approach that includes prevention.

We live in a world between expectation and reality – and our goal as providers is to help ourselves and our patients anticipate problems and provide solutions. A smoker may have expectations of invincibility. Like many of you, I have succeeded most often in getting the person to quit by appealing to the vanity of the smoker by pointing out the accumulated wrinkles if he or she persists. If that method works, it is a success!

Time's arrow only moves in one direction – forward – and chronological aging takes a toll on all of us, especially visible on the most recognizable features of our facial skin. A rising tide of boomers are arriving daily at the shores of older age and demanding more help, including prevention of skin problems.

Much can be done to prevent the disfiguring effects brought on by the abuse of sun, nicotine and alcohol, excess weight, mobility and exercise difficulties, dysfunctional nutrition, improper hygiene, lack of immunizations, poor reading and comprehension skills, inadequate cosmetic repair, and many other problems. Preventive dermatology focuses on ways we can minimize skin problems, and maximize and enjoy the time we have been given.

We have highly effective sunscreens, a plethora of information about skin care on the internet, and more prevention and treatment modalities than ever before. But even the most informed patients need guidance, and that's why you need the information included in this book. I hope you share this information with your colleagues and patients, and this first book on prevention in dermatology is a springboard for many more books, ideas, and discussions to improve the quality of our lives.

Tampa, FL   Dr. Robert A. Norman

Contents

Alistair Mackenzie Library
Wishaw General Hospital
50 Netherton Street
Wishaw
ML2 0DP

Contributors

Susan R. Adams Department of Health Science (Addiction Studies), University of Central Arkansas, Conway, AR, USA

Hillary E. Baldwin Department of Dermatology, SUNY – Brooklyn, Brooklyn, NY, USA

Michelle C. Duhaney Department of Family Medicine, Broward General Medical Centre, Fort Lauderdale, FL, USA

Cynthia A. Fleck, The American Academy of Wound Management (AAWM), Washington, DC, USA and
The Association for the Advancement of Wound Care (AAWC), St. Louis, MO, USA and Clinical Marketing, Medline Industries, Inc., St. Louis, MO, USA

Michael R. Hinckley Department of Dermatology, Wake Forest University Baptist Medical Center, Winston-Salem, NC, USA

Jina P. Lewallen Department of Geriatrics, University of Arkansas for Medical Sciences, Little Rock, AR, USA

Robert A. Norman Nova Southeastern University, Ft. Lauderdale, FL, USA and Private Practice, Tampa, FL, USA

Max J. Rappaport 4th Year Medical Student, LECOM, Bradenton, FL, USA

Nana Smith Department of Dermatology, University of Rochester, Rochester, NY, USA

Francisco A. Tausk Department of Dermatology, University of Rochester, Rochester, NY, USA

Carolyn Lazaro Turturro Graduate Gerontology Program, School of Social Work, University of Arkansas at Little Rock, Little Rock, AR, USA

Angelo Turturro Graduate Gerontology Program, School of Social Work, University of Arkansas at Little Rock, Little Rock, AR, USA

Stress, Relaxation, and General Well-Being

1

Nana Smith and Francisco A. Tausk

Your pain is the breaking of the shell that encloses your understanding. ... It is the bitter potion by which the physician within you heals your sick self. Therefore trust the physician, and drink his remedy in silence and tranquility...

From The Prophet, Khalil Gibran

We instinctively understand that, in general, stress is an uncomfortable and deleterious physical and emotional state. However, it is often difficult to recognize and control. In dermatology, stress can be both a consequence and an instigator of disease. This chapter will explore (1) definitions of stress, (2) the interplay between stress and the skin, and (3) various stress-reducing modalities.

1.1 Stress

Stress encompasses a myriad of emotional and physical triggers which have a taxing effect on our bodies. Stress can be acute or chronic. As humans, we are well adapted to acute stress. Imagine the changes in our predecessors' heart rate and blood flow in response to the proximity of a predator. However, it could be argued that the concept of chronic stress is a creation of the modern world. Our ability to adapt to chronic stress is not necessarily innate and requires a much more creative and active approach.

Stress can be considered as a disruption of balance which triggers various adaptive responses. Hans Selye, a 1930s endocrinologist, coined the term *stress* and defined it in terms of the General Adaptation Syndrome. Throughout his career he performed various experiments which showed that animals respond to stress in three stages. In the General Adaption Syndrome, the first stage is alarm. The physiology of this stage is well-understood and represents an acute response to stress. The sympathetic nervous system is activated, releasing catecholamines (CA) such as epinephrine and norepinephrine. This is the *fight-or-flight* response which causes blood to flow toward large muscular groups and away from the gastrointestinal system, the skin, and other organs. Walter Cannon, who in the 1920s first coined the term "fight or flight"[1] described the responses of the sympathetic nervous system and adrenal gland to environmental stressors.[2] The hypothalamic-pituitary-adrenal (HPA) axis is also stimulated, which releases hormones such as cortisol. Resistance is the second stage. Here the body's coping resources are gradually diminished. In the final, exhaustion stage, the resources are depleted and the subject is unable to maintain homeostasis. Interestingly, the fight-or-flight response may now briefly reappear. However, with continued stressors, the adrenal gland and the immune system are sufficiently taxed and illnesses begin to manifest. This is analogous to a state of chronic stress.

The term *allostasis* refers to the balance between stressors and coping mechanisms; it is the ability to adapt to maintain balance and stability. This is a slightly different framework for stress than that defined by Seyle.[3] Allostasis is different from homeostasis in that homeostasis is concerned with minute-to-minute

N. Smith (✉)
Department of Dermatology,
University of Rochester,
Rochester, NY, USA
e-mail: nananamibia_smith@urmc.rochester.edu

R.A. Norman (ed.), *Common Treatments in Preventive Dermatology*,
DOI 10.1007/978-0-85729-853-9_1, © Springer-Verlag London Limited 2012

regulation of bodily functions in a very narrow range whereas in allostasis the range is much wider. McEwen views the consequences of chronic stress as a type of *allostatic load* which can build up and lead to disease. In the ideal situation, a person is presented with a stressor, the body compensates by initiating certain stress responses, and when the stressor is gone, the stress response is shut off. In this situation, there is little allostatic load. Conditions in which allostatic load can build up include frequent stressor over time, lack of adaptation to stressors (decreased response to stressors over time), inability to shut down a stress response, and inadequate initial response which leads to compensations by other stress responses.[4]

Acute and chronic stresses have different effects on our bodies. The effects are seen in the cardiovascular and endocrine/metabolic systems, the brain, and the immune system.

1.2 Stress, Immune Function, and the Skin

There is a complex interplay between stressors, the central nervous system, the endocrine system, immune function, and the skin. The HPA axis is stimulated by signals which are processed in the hypothalamus and the brain stem (locus coeruleus [LC]). In response to these stressors, the hypothalamus secretes corticotrophin-releasing hormone (CRH). From the hypothalamus, CRH-containing neurons communicate with the brain stem and spinal cord. CRH release further activates the HPA axis by causing the release of peptides from the pituitary. The peptides, such as adrenocorticotropic hormone (ACTH), enkephalins, and endorphins, are produced by the differential cleavage of pro-opiomelanocortin (POMC). ACTH induces release of glucocorticoids (GC) such as cortisol from the adrenal cortex. Activation of the noradrenergic pathways by CRH-containing neurons results in secretion of norepinephrine (NE) by the sympathetic nervous system and release of NE and epinephrine (EPI) from the adrenal medulla. These are called CA. The activation of the sympathetic nervous system and the adrenal cortex and the subsequent release of hormones and neurotransmitters have significant effects on the immune system (Fig. 1.1).

In general, Th1-derived cytokines (IFN-α, IL-2) are considered proinflammatory whereas Th2-derived cytokines (IL-4, IL-5, IL-10) are considered anti-inflammatory. Both GCs and CAs have the ability to create a shift toward the Th2 pathway by up-regulating Th2-cytokine production and also by suppressing APC production of IL-12 and Th1 cytokine synthesis[5] (Fig. 1.1). APC-derived IL-12 is one of the main inducers of Th1 cytokine synthesis.[6] Therefore, chronic stress is essentially immunosuppressive. Furthermore, immune challenges such as bacterial infections can result in the release of bacterial lipopolysaccharides

---

Fig. 1.1 The hypothalamic-pituitary-adrenal (HPA) axis and immunity. The identification of an external perceived stressor by the brain results in the activation of the paraventricular nucleus of the hypothalamus and the closely interconnected locus coeruleus. CRF is secreted from the hypothalamus and transported through the portal circulation to the pituitary, where it induces the release of ACTH from the anterior pituitary into the general circulation. The effect of this molecule results in the secretion of glucocorticosteroids and to a lesser extent CA from the adrenal gland. Cortisol will act as a negative feedback on the hypothalamus, inhibiting the release of CRF. The cells of the locus coeruleus have a rich neuronal connection with the PVN, and activate the sympathetic system which results in the secretion of epinephrine and norepinephrine. Both the cathecholamines and cortisol have a potent effect on the immune system. They modulate antigen presenting cells and macrophages inhibiting their activity and the production of IL-12 and IL-18, and they mediate the differentiation of naïve T helper cells towards the TH2 constellation, in detriment of the development of TH1 mediated immunity. This results in tilting the balance towards humoral immunity by increasing the production of IL-4, IL-5, and IL-13, which activate B-cells, mast cells, and eosinophils, increasing the allergic inflammatory response. The chronic dampening of cell-mediated immunity could result in an impaired ability to confront effectively the development of infectious or tumoral insults. On the other hand, internal stressors are exemplified here by bacterial infections. The released bacterial lipopolysaccharides (LPS) bind to toll-like receptors on macrophages, and through NFκB induce the production of IL-1 and IL-6. These cytokines are able to cross the blood–brain barrier and reach the hypothalamus, where they stimulate the secretion of CRF, initiating the activation of the HPA axis. In this manner, infections have the potential to shift the immune balance favoring the humoral TH2 mediated response. Diseases that involve this arm of the immune system such as autoimmune or allergic diseases would deteriorate during the presence of stressors of the internal as well as external kind. Stimulation (*straight arrows*). Inhibition (*broken arrows*) (Reproduced with permission from Harth et al.[103])

(LPS) which induces the nuclear factor (NF) kb mediated secretion of IL-1 and IL-6. These cytokines are responsible for fatigue, somnolence, and fever. These cytokines (IL-1, IL-6) stimulate the hypothalamic stress response in a positive feedback loop (Fig. 1.1). One main mechanism for the ability of GCs to suppress APCs is by inhibiting the costimulatory molecules necessary for T cell activation. GCs also decrease the ability of neutrophils to find sites of inflammation (decreased chemotaxis) and to attach to vascular endothelium and extravasate into the tissue.

The skin itself is a major source of central neuroendocrine stress mediators and has fully active peripheral equivalents of central stress responses systems. For example, skin cells produce a variety of neuropeptides, hormones, and neurotransmitters which have been implicated in modulating immune function in the skin, communicating with the hypothalamus, and playing a role in the development of skin diseases. The brain can affect inflammatory conditions in the skin but stimuli received by the skin can also influence the immune, endocrine, and nervous systems.[7]

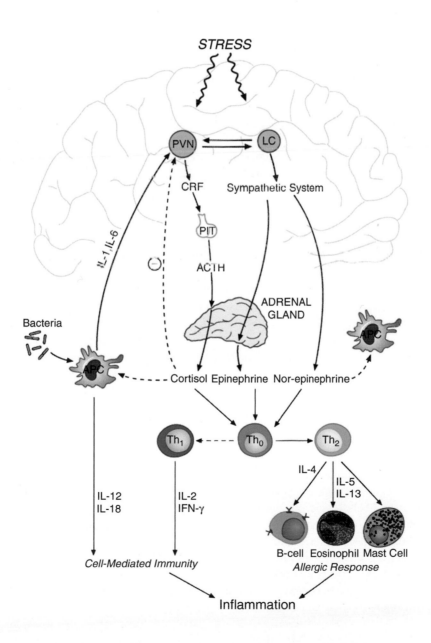

Stress decreases wound-healing capacities. Kiecolt-Glaser et al. found that in normal, healthy dental students, the time to heal a mucosal wound was approximately 3 days slower at the time of examination.[8] They also showed that married couples with hostile interactions had impaired wound healing compared to happier couples. These findings may be explained by the effects of stress on matrix metalloproteinases (MMPs) and the tissue inhibitors of metalloproteinases (TIMPs).[9, 10] Tausk et al. investigated the effects of stress in mice induced by the smell of fox urine (a natural predator). Mice exposed to stress showed delayed wound healing compared to control mice (unpublished data).

As most dermatologists have witnessed from their patients, skin disease is often worsened or initiated by stressful situations. Patients even associate conditions that have not been described in the literature as being stress-associated with increased stress in their lives. The stressor need not be emotional in nature; we are well aware of dermatologic conditions associated with recent illness, a type of physical stress. Emotional stressors have been associated with the development or worsening of a variety of dermatologic diseases including acne, vitiligo, alopecia areata, lichen planus, seborrheic dermatitis, telogen effluvium, herpes simplex infections, pemphigus, urticaria, psoriasis, angioedema atopic dermatitis, hyperhidrosis, neurotic excoriations, warts, cysts, and more.[11–18]

Stress has been reported to both precede the onset of psoriasis[19] and to trigger flares.[20, 21] The observation that led to further study of psoriasis and stress involved psoriasis patients who have undergone physical trauma. In some cases, where there was traumatic disconnection of sensory nerves, the psoriatic skin in the innervated areas resolved. When the fibers regenerated and sensitivity returned, the psoriatic plaques returned. It was hypothesized that local neuropeptides where responsible for the persistence of psoriatic plaques. It was later discovered that not only do psoriatic plaques have different content of neuropeptides such as SP (substance P), VIP (vasoactive intestinal peptide), CGRP(calcitonin gene-related protein), and NGF (nerve growth factor) but the density of nerve fibers in the plaques is elevated.[22–25] Increased levels of NGF causes T cell and keratinocyte proliferation, mast cell degranulation, and memory T cell chemotaxis, which are all features seen in psoriasis.[26–28] The HPA axis in psoriasis patients also exhibits an insufficient production of cortisol in the face of experimental stressors.[29, 30]

In atopic dermatitis, stress can also worsen the existing disease and stimulate flares.[31, 32] In experimental studies, stress has been found to interfere with the barrier function of the skin.[33] When the straum corneum is unable to recover from transepidermal water loss, the barrier is disrupted, inviting various infectious agents and allergens to initiate a disease flare.[34] Another explanation for the connection between stress and atopic dermatitis is that, much as in psoriasis, patients with this disease have an insufficient HPA axis response to stress.[35–37] Interestingly, the circulating leukocytes in patients with atopic dermatitis have a higher number of GC receptors than control patients. Therefore, and perhaps in compensation for a blunted HPA response, when immune cells are exposed to even a small amount of cortisol produced by stress they are hyperactive along the cortisol-induced Th2 pathway.[38] This is detrimental, as IL-4 and IL-10 activate mast cells, eosinophils, and IgE production which further worsens atopic dermatitis. The worsening of atopic dermatitis in the face of stress may also be, in part, caused by the effects of epinephrine.[39]

Episodes of urticaria, especially adrenergic urticaria, have been associated with stressful events. Again, the cortisol-induced upregulation of Th2 cytokines, leading to the activation and degranulation of mast cells could explain this phenomenon[40] as well as the fact that mast cell CRH receptors[41] are upregulated under stress.

Stress also plays a role in infections of the skin including those bacterial, viral, and fungal in nature.[42–46] In rats, stressed by restraining them, HSV is reactivated in the dorsal root ganglion. Epidemiologic studies have found that in humans it is chronic, not necessarily acute stress which is associated with more frequent outbreaks.[46, 47] Various stress-reducing techniques have been shown to reduce outbreak frequency.[48]

In both human and animal studies, stress has been linked to malignancy, perhaps by suppressing lymphocyte and especially natural killer (NK) cell activity.[49–62]

Parker et al. reported findings linking stress to skin cancer in mice.[63] Two groups of mice were exposed to UV light; one group was stressed by the smell of a predator and the other group was not. The stressed group developed squamous cell carcinomas (SCCs) significantly earlier than the nonstressed group (SCC at week 8 vs. week 21, $p < 0.05$). This observation was confirmed by another group.[64] Stress-reducing interventions have shown a survival benefit for patients with malignancies.[65] For example, patients with metastatic melanoma had an increased 6-year survival rate when a stress-reducing and psychological intervention was made.[66] Again, this may be linked to altered NK function under stressful situations.[67] In other studies, the cytotoxic function of the lymphocytes in older adults and in immunocompetent medical students was altered by chronic stress; relaxation training increased this cytotoxic function.[68] Other mice models have shown that chronic stress suppresses lymphocyte proliferation, increases metastases risk and growth of the primary tumor.[69–71]

1.3 Epidemiology

Use of various stress-reducing modalities for skin disease is common among dermatologic patients throughout the world.[72]

A study performed in Leeds and South Wales in the United Kingdom investigated the use of complementary and alternative medicine (CAM) among patients presenting to an outpatient dermatology clinic. Three hundred and two completed questionnaires in Leeds and 415 in South Wales revealed that about 20% of Leeds patients and 5% of South Wales patients used aromatherapy. Faith or spiritual healing was used in about 10% in each group. Hypnotherapy was used in approximately 10% of Leeds patients and 5% of South Wales patients. Massage was used by around 15% of Leeds patients.[73] Researchers elsewhere conducted 109 face-to-face interviews of patients referred to contact dermatitis clinic and found that aromatherapy was used by 18%.[74] A German study conducted a validated questionnaire in 1,288 patients; 73 patients with atopic dermatitis under conventional therapy and 59 patients under alternative-medical therapy. In the alternative therapy group 65% used autogenic training and 43% used relaxation procedures for their skin disease. The numbers were 29 and 13% respectively for the conventional group.[75] A study of 198 patients from the dermatology clinic at Show Chwan Memorial Hosp in Changhua City, Taiwan found that aromatherapy (4.6%), Qi-gong/Tai-Chi/yoga (r%), religion (1.5%), and meditation/hypnosis (0.5%) were used.[76] A self-administered questionnaire from 70 patients with atopic dermatitis referred to the university clinic at Oregon Health and Science University revealed that hypnosis (10.3%), massage (10.3%), and biofeedback (3.4%) were commonly used.[77]

1.4 Stress-Reducing Modalities

In the realm of CAM, it is the mind–body interventions that have the most obvious implications for stress reduction. Use of mind–body interventions by the general American public is common (though not necessarily among dermatology patients). In 2002, mind–body techniques, including relaxation, meditation, guided imagery, biofeedback, and hypnosis were used by about 17% of the adult US population. Prayer was used by 45% of the population for health reasons.[78]

These modalities have shown their use in a variety of conditions: from coronary artery disease[79] and pain control[80, 81] to managing the symptoms of cancer and the side effects of its treatment.[82–84]

There are a multitude of case reports, case series, and some clinical trials suggesting that various mind–body interventions are useful in dermatologic conditions. The findings which relate to dermatology will be presented at the end of each of the following sections where appropriate. We will now look more closely into various stress-reducing techniques which may be helpful for people with skin disease.

1.4.1 Yoga

Yoga is a spiritual practice which incorporates physical activity (breathing exercises and poses or postures) and meditation to create a connection between the mind and body.[85] It has been used in India for over 5,000 years as a system of healing and a framework for how to live one's life and obtain spiritual enlightenment. In the West, however, it grew popular as a form of exercise. Yoga was first introduced to the American society in the late nineteenth century by Swami Vivekananda. He believed that India had an abundance of spiritual wealth and that yoga could help those in Western societies to achieve spiritual well-being. Most yoga classes consist of a combination of physical exercises, breathing exercises, chanting, and meditation. Yoga may improve resistance to psychological stress, decrease feelings of bodily self-objectification, and promote a feeling of wholeness, balance, and well-being.[85, 86]

According to a survey by the National Center for CAM, yoga was the fifth most commonly used CAM therapy (2.8%) in the United States during 2002.[78] It is thought by its practitioners to prevent specific diseases by keeping "energy meridians" open and "life energy" (*Prana*) freely flowing. Yoga is usually performed in group classes. Sessions are conducted at least once a week and for approximately 45 min. Yoga has been used to lower blood pressure, reduce stress, and improve coordination, flexibility, concentration, sleep, and digestion. It has also been used as supplementary therapy for such diverse conditions as cancer, diabetes, asthma, AIDS, and irritable bowel syndrome.[87]

There are many different styles of yoga; each has a particular emphasis.

Hatha is a term that can encompass many of the physical types of yoga. It is slow-paced and gentle and is a good introduction to the basic yoga poses. *Vinyasa*, which means breath-synchronized movement, is a more vigorous style in which various poses (sun salutations) are connected to certain breathing techniques. *Ashtanga*, or power yoga is not recommended for beginning students. This is an intense, fast-paced style in which the poses are sequentially performed leading to a fluid movement from one pose to the other. *Iyengar* yoga is focused on bodily alignment and is interested in the details of each posture. The poses are typically held much longer than in other styles and props such as blankets, blocks, and straps are also used. This is a good style for beginners. *Bikram* yoga or hot yoga is practiced in a 95–100°room, which creates a sauna-like effect that is thought to be cleansing and good for the muscles. *Anusara* combines an emphasis on alignment with the belief that there is intrinsic goodness in all beings. These classes are good for students of differing abilities and are very calming. *Kundalini* is an energizing form of yoga which is aimed at freeing "dormant spiritual energy" at the base of the spine and allowing it to move upwards. *Jivamukti* yoga is athletic, physically challenging but highly meditative. The focus is on fitness. Integral yoga is a gentle *Hatha* style which follows the teachings of Sri Swami Sachidananda, who came to the United States in the 1960s. It is aimed at helping people integrate yoga's teachings into everyday life. *Sivananda* is a traditional, more lifestyle approach to yoga. The class structure is rigid and is based on five principles: proper exercise, proper breathing, proper relaxation, proper diet (vegetarian), and positive thinking and meditation. *Kripalu* yoga is focused on healing. It is great for beginning students and teaches inner focus and meditation, focus on alignment, breath, and presence of consciousness. Integrative yoga was designed for medical and main-

stream wellness settings (hospitals and rehab). It involves gentle postures, guided imagery, and breathing techniques for treating specific health issues. It emphasizes holistic healing.

1.4.2 Deep Breathing

Deep breathing is the act of breathing deep into your lungs by expanding your diaphragm rather than breathing shallowly by expanding your rib cage. It is also called diaphragmatic breathing, abdominal breathing, or belly breathing. When you breathe deeply your abdominal wall expands rather contracts. It is often used for hyperventilation and anxiety. To perform diaphragmatic breathing one should sit or lie wearing loose comfortable clothing. One hand is placed on the chest and one on the abdomen. Inhale through the nose or pursed lips. During inhalation, the abdomen should expand or press outward, the chest should not. Slowly exhale through pursed lips and then rest and repeat. The inhalation and exhalation times should be about equal. This method of stress reduction may be difficult for people with diaphragmatic dysfunction from various respiratory or neuromuscular conditions.

1.4.3 Tai Chi

Tai chi originated in China as a martial art. Over time, people also began to use it for health purposes. Tai chi incorporates a series of exercises that mimic the movements of certain animals with concepts of flexibility and meditation. The body moves slowly and gently, while the person is breathing deeply and meditating. Tai Chi practitioners believe that tai chi helps the flow of "vital energy" called *qi*. One can practice alone or in a group. Many movements are named for animals or birds, such as "White Crane Spreads Its Wings." The simplest styles of tai chi incorporate 13 movements into a routine, but more complex routine can be learned. The entire body is always in motion as one movement flows into another. The upper body is kept upright and it is important to concentrate and not be distracted. Breathing should be deep, relaxed, and focused. People practice tai chi for a variety of health purposes including pain control, stress reduction, insomnia, enhancing coordination, flexibility and balance, and overall well-being. Tai chi is practiced by many people in China, even in hospitals and clinics. It is especially beneficial for the elderly.

1.4.4　Progressive Relaxation

Progressive muscle relaxation was developed by an American physician Edmund Jacobson in the early 1920s as a stress reduction technique. It remains popular with modern physical therapists. The goal is to reduce anxiety and the effects of stress of the musculature. Jacobson found that the technique is also effective against ulcers, insomnia, and hypertension. Progressive relaxation is similar to autogenic training which is a form of self-hypnosis. The technique involves progressively tensing and then relaxing every consciously controlled muscle group until the entire body is relaxed; the sequence usually goes from head to foot. It is best done lying down on the floor or a bed.

1.4.5　Aromatherapy

Aromatherapy is the use of plant-derived essential oils as a form of supportive care to improve quality of life and reduce stress and anxiety. Fragrant oils have been used for health purposes for thousands of years and in a variety of cultures. Essential oils (or volatile oils) are derived from various parts of the plant (leaves, bark, peel) and are usually extracted using alcohol.

They are very concentrated. Aromatherapy likely works through smell receptors in the nose communicating with the brain's limbic system and altering mood and emotions. The volatile oils are either inhaled by using a diffuser, or applied topically (usually in a diluted form) as part of a massage, poultice, or bath. Aromatherapy may improve quality of life in patients with cancer with regard to reducing side effects such as nausea, anxiety, and insomnia. Safety testing on essential oils shows few side effects when they are used as directed. Some essential oils have been approved as ingredients in food and are classified as GRAS (generally recognized as safe) by the US Food and Drug Administration. However, allergic contact or irritant dermatitis may occur in aromatherapists or in patients

using aromatherapy, especially with long periods of skin contact. Photosensitivity may develop when citrus or other oils are applied to the skin before sun exposure. Lavender and tea tree oils have been found to have hormone-like effects similar to estrogen and also block or decrease the effect of androgens. Applying lavender and tea tree oils to the skin over a long period of time has been linked to gynecomastia in prepubescent boys. Essential oils with aldehyde or phenols structures especially cause an irritant dermatitis. Oils with ketone derivatives can cause neurotoxicity in epileptics, pregnant women, and babies. Sassafras oil and calamus oil have been shown to be carcinogenic.[88, 89]

Stevensen reviewed the dermatologic applications of various essential oils. Some of the antiseptic oils were geranium, petitgrain, winter savory, and tea tree oil. Juniper berry has anti-inflammatory properties whereas frankincense is an immunostimulant. French lavender is useful for burns, cajeput for genital herpes, and chamomile and lavender are good for stress reduction.[88]

Bensouilah also reviewed the use of aromatherapy in psoriatic patients to reduce disease severity and symptoms and to increase quality of life. Several anti-inflammatory oils were listed which may be helpful in psoriasis including *achillea millefolium*, borage oil, evening primrose oil, sweet almond oil, jojoba wax, tamanu oil (for the scalp especially), calendula, and avocado oil.[89]

When mice with experimental contact hypersensitivity were exposed to terpinyl acetate (which has a herbal lavender woody smell) and valerian oil in the presence of stress, the contact hypersensitivity worsened. The theory is that if stress is immunosuppressive, which would mute a contact dermatitis, stress reduction (via pleasant scents) would attenuate some of this immunosuppression and a more florid skin response would be seen. Valerian oil was also found to down-regulate stress-induced plasma corticosterone levels in the mice.[90] Another study in mice suggested that the smell of tuberose, lemon, oakmoss, and labdanum reduces some of the immunologic effects of high-pressure-induced stress.[91] Finally, in human volunteers, the smell of lavender and rosemary decreased saliva cortisol and increased free radical scavenging activity.[92]

A randomized controlled double blind trial of aromatherapy for alopecia areata was performed in 86 patients in an outpatient setting. Patients were randomized to massaged thyme, rosemary, lavender, and cedarwood oil mixed in carrier oils (jojoba and grape-seed) vs. the carrier oils alone. These oils were massaged onto the scalp daily for 7 months and results were evaluated at 3 and 7 months in terms of dermotologist-evaluated photographs and computer analysis of severity. Forty-four percent of patients in the aromatherapy group vs. 15% of patients in the control group showed improvement at the end of the trial ($p > 0.008$).[93]

1.4.6 Massage

Massage therapy refers to a group of practices and techniques involving pressing, rubbing, and manipulation of the muscles and other soft tissues of the body. Most often the hands and fingers are used but forearms, elbows, feet, hot stones, and other tools are sometimes used. Some examples are Swedish massage, deep tissue massage, and shiatsu massage. A 2002 national survey on Americans' use of CAM (published in 2004) found that 5% of the 31,000 participants had used massage therapy in the preceding 12 months, and 9.3% had ever used it.[78] People use massage for a variety of reasons including pain relief, rehabilitation, stress reduction, and general well-being. Patients with a deep vein thrombosis, bleeding disorders or on anticoagulation, peripheral vascular disease, osteoporosis or recent fracture, tumors, open or healing wounds, neuropathy, or myopathies should consult their physician before receiving massage.

In addition to providing stress reduction, massage may be beneficial in certain dermatologic conditions for other reasons. For example, emollients may be more effectively applied by massage in patients with atopic dermatitis, psoriasis, other dermatitic conditions, and icthiosis. Massage is often used as an adjuvant to compression stockings in lymphedema clinics. There is some theoretic suggestion that massage may help prevent fibrosis which may be useful in combination with conventional therapies for morphea and other fibrotic disorders. In general, touching the skin of our patients communicates lack of repulsion and judgment which is incredibly important in conditions like psoriasis which cause profound feelings of stigma and alienation.

1.4.7 Mindfulness Meditation

Meditation refers to a group of techniques, the goal of which is to enhance health and wellness through the quiet focusing attention and maintenance of an open mind. Most time meditation involves a specific posture. People who practice meditation can often increase relaxation, calmness, and mental balance and enhance coping. Research using functional magnetic resonance imaging (fMRI) suggests that the areas of the brain involved in paying attention and in the control of the autonomic nervous system are stimulated during meditation. A large national survey on Americans' use of CAM, found that nearly 8% of the participants had used meditation specifically for health reasons during the year before the survey.[78] Mindfulness meditation has its origins in Buddhism. The concept is that one is fully present during the meditation process; this involves being "mindful" or aware of thoughts, emotions, and physical feelings (including breath), whatever they may be.

Gaston et al. performed a randomized, controlled trial to evaluate the efficacy of meditation as an adjunctive treatment for scalp psoriasis. For 20 weeks, 24 subjects were randomly allocated to one of four groups: meditation, meditation and imagery, waiting list for treatment, and a treatment-free control. Eighteen subjects completed the trial. The meditation group did home meditation for 30 min daily. Subjects were allowed to continue their conventional psoriasis medications. The investigators used a blinded clinical severity score consisting of thickness, erythema, and scale and surface area. Using a Spearman's coefficient, the group was measuring the relationship over time between psoriasis and stress. The investigators found a significant difference between meditation vs. the control groups for treatment of psoriasis ($r > 0.30, p < 0.01$), with no impact of imagery. The clinical assessment also strongly supported this finding.[94]

Kabat, Zinn, et al. performed a controlled trial with two independent randomization steps: randomization into ultraviolet B (UVB) vs. psoralen and ultraviolet A (PUVA) cohorts and randomization into use of a mindfulness-based stress reduction audiotape during light therapy vs. no audiotape.[94] Patients received either UVB or PUVA therapy three times weekly until their psoriasis cleared or they dropped out of the study. During their light therapy, half of the subjects listened to tapes that encouraged being mindful of breathing, of body sensation, of ambient sounds, thoughts, and feelings and encouraged visualization of UV light slowing down the division of skin cells. The other half (control) received light therapy in silence. Thirty-seven subjects with moderate to severe psoriasis participated in the study. Their rate of psoriatic lesion clearing was assessed on four occasions in three independent ways: directly by unblinded clinic nurses, directly by blinded physicians, and indirectly via lesion photographs by blinded physicians. Time to first response, time to turning point, and time to halfway clearing were measured. In the UVB group there was a significantly shorter time to turning point and time to halfway clearing compared to controls ($p > 0.005$, 0.002, respectively). In the PUVA group there was no significant difference between groups. Using Cox-proportional hazards regression models which adjust for confounding factors such as years with psoriasis and initial psychological state, estimated response time-to-clearance curves were constructed. These estimated curves showed a significantly shorter time-to-clearance between mindfulness tape and no mindfulness tape groups.[95]

1.4.8 Biofeedback

Biofeedback is a procedure which provides the subject with feedback about certain bodily functions with the assistance of certain instruments. It provides a sort of mirror for various types of biological information. One is connected to a machine that monitors heart beat, muscle tone, skin temperature or resistance, and electric potential of the brain (EEG) for instance. The subject receives information about the activity level of those functions in the form of visual or auditory signals. The goal is to consciously control these functions to reach a desired state (i.e., reduced skin temperature in psoriasis). The most common forms of biofeedback are galvanic skin response, electromyographic biofeedback, thermal biofeedback, and electroencephalographic rhythm biofeedback. The electromyographic biofeedback (which measures variations in muscle electric potential) is best for anxiety states. Two phases are usually performed. There is a relaxation phase in which the practitioner gathers information about the patient's life experiences, difficulties relaxing, and various images, thoughts, or sensations. The technical phase is when the therapist takes measurements and helps the patient overcome obstacles to relaxation. Usually 10–20 sessions are needed, with 1–2/week. Patients are encouraged to practice at home for 20 min a day using elementary portable instruments. The goal

is that control of the function becomes automatic such that the subject can reproduce it in stressful situations.[96] The most reasonable application in dermatology would be for neurodermatitis and related disorders (trichotillomania) and for pruritis.

Keinan et al. treated 32 subjects in a 3-month randomized, double-blind, controlled trial in which subjects were divided into three groups. One group was trained to do biofeedback and relaxation techniques, one relaxation only and the third group received no treatment. Efficacy was evaluated by a six-point symptom severity scale which ranged from *no symptoms* to *very severe symptoms* and by a symptom improvement scale, a nine-point scale ranging from *complete remission* to *extreme worsening*. No significant changes in symptom severity scale or symptom improvement scale were found.[97]

Biofeedback has also been reported to have efficacy in hyperhidrosis and Raynaud's disease.

1.4.9 Autogenic Training

Autogenic training is a form of self-hypnosis and relaxation which is usually used for stress control. Stewart and Thomas treated 18 adults with extensive atopic dermatitis with hypnotherapy, relaxation, and stress management. During the hypnotherapy patients received direct suggestions for nonscratching behavior, skin comfort and coolness, and ego strengthening. Patients also received instructions on self-hypnosis. In this non-randomized controlled clinical trial, significant reductions in itching, scratching, sleep disturbance, and tension were found compared to the control group. Use of topical steroids decreased by 60% at 16 weeks.[98]

1.4.10 Hypnosis

Hypnosis was initially described in the late eighteenth century by Franz Anton Mesmer and was further developed by Milton Erickson in modern times. It is an altered state of consciousness in which the suggestions from someone else, the environment, or from oneself, allow the imagination to create a vivid reality. People innately have different levels of suggestiveness; in other words, people who are highly suggestible are more likely to benefit from hypnosis. It is difficult to predict a person's level of suggestiveness.

Many case reports of dermatologic conditions responding to hypnosis have been published.[94] These include clearing of congenital ichthyosiform erythroderma of Brocq, erythromelalgia, herpes simplex, acne excoriee, alopecia areata, trichotillomania, neurodermatitis, furuncles, rosacea, vitiligo, and others. There have been case series of the efficacy of hypnosis for urticaria. Nonrandomized controlled trials exist for atopic dermatitis and, for verruca vulgaris, psoriasis and relaxation during procedures, there have been randomized controlled trials. Controlled studies using direct suggestion in hypnosis (DSIH) for warts show success rates between 27% and 55%. Children respond especially well.[99]

Tausk and Whitmore used hypnosis to treat psoriasis in a randomized, controlled, single-blind, 3-month study. Eleven patients with mild-to-moderate stable psoriasis were randomized to one of two groups: hypnosis with active suggestion or neutral hypnosis. In the active treatment, group subjects were asked to image the conventional therapy which they believed to be most effective for their psoriasis. Only subjects who were identified as being highly or moderately suggestible were included in the study. Subjects were treated with weekly hypnosis sessions for 3 months according to the treatment group; then the investigator was unblinded and both groups received active suggestion hypnosis for 3 more months. Psoriasis severity was assessed using the Psoriasis Area and Severity Index (PASI) and was performed by a different, blinded investigator. Results showed that highly suggestible individuals vs. moderately suggestible individuals had a significant improvement in psoriasis severity ($p < 0.05$).[100]

1.4.11 QI Gong/Reiki/Healing Touch

Energy medicine is a CAM modality that deals with energy fields of two types: veritable and putative. The veritable energies are those that can be measured; they use vibrations, electromagnetic forces, visible light, and monochromatic radiation (i.e., LASER) for example. Putative energy cannot be measured. CAM modalities which claim to alter this subtle, immeasurable energy are reiki, qi gong, and healing touch.

Qi gong is practiced commonly in clinics and hospitals of China. It is a branch of traditional Chinese medicine which is aimed at restoring balance and the

free flow of qi or life energy. Reiki is a similar practice that originated in Japan. Therapeutic touch is perhaps the Western equivalent of the prior two modalities. All three involve movement of the practitioner's hands over the patient's body to sense and ultimately manipulate energy throughout the body.

The evidence for these modalities is mixed and sparse. However, to the extent that they reduce stress, reiki, qi gong, and healing touch may be useful in dermatology patients.

1.4.12 Prayer

Particularly devastating dermatologic conditions have the potential to alter our patients' sense of spiritual well-being. Sometimes a sense of spirituality may allow a patient to better cope with a particular condition or diagnosis, other times patients feel a sense of divine punishment from their skin condition. It is important to know the role that spirituality plays in our patients' lives, to the extent that we can support any positive attributes it may add to conventional management. If the patient obtains emotional support from his/her spirituality it would be appropriate to encourage patients to speak with a chaplain, clergy member, or spiritual leader regarding the condition. Dermatologists, and any physician, should respectfully support the patient's use of spirituality to cope with their disease. If one feels comfortable, it is appropriate to both pray for and with patients when they are facing difficult times or decisions.[101]

In an Austrian study, 215 patients with melanoma were interviewed about their interests in CAM and reasons for pursuing this. More than half had an interest in nonconventional therapies. Interested subjects had a more active coping style, a tendency toward religiousness, and need to search for personal meaning in their disease than noninterested subjects. They also believed that they were receiving less emotional support from their physicians than the other group and expressed interest in getting more of such support.[102]

1.5 Conclusion

As dermatologists, we have no less of an obligation to practice in the context of a bio-psycho-social model than other physicians. We should make it a habit to ask our patients about their stress levels and to what extent it contributes to their skin disease. It is also important to have practical advice to offer patients in terms of stress reduction techniques. To the extent of our control, the office setting and the personal experiences patients encounter in the clinic should be relaxing and promoting of the healing process. Also, in order to effective carry out our responsibilities as physicians, each of us should frequently monitor and control the stress in our own lives so that optimal care of our patients is not compromised.

References

1. Cannon WB. *The Wisdom of the Body*. New York: Norton; 1932
2. Selye H. *The Stress of Life*. New York: McGraw-Hill; 1956
3. Sterling P, Eyer J. Allostasis: a new paradigm to explain arousal pathology. In: Fisher S, Reason J, eds. *Handbook of Life Stress, Cognition and Health*. New York: John Wiley; 1988:629–649
4. McEwen BS. Protective and damaging effects of stress mediators. Seminars in Medicine of the Beth Israel Deaconess Medical Center. *N Engl J Med*. 1998;338(3):171–179
5. Elenkov IJ, Chrousos GP. Stress hormones, Th1/Th2 patterns, pro/anti-inflammatory cytokines and susceptibility to disease. *Trends Endocrinol Metab*. 1999;10(9):359–368
6. Trinchieri G. Interleukin-12 and the regulation of innate resistance and adaptive immunity. *Nat Rev* 2003;3(2):133–146
7. Marucha PT, Kiecolt-Glaser JK, Favagehi M. Mucosal wound healing is impaired by examination stress. *Psychosom Med*. 1998;60(3):362–365
8. Stamenkovic I. Extracellular matrix remodelling: the role of matrix metalloproteinases. *J Pathol*. 2003;200(4):448–464
9. Yang EV, Bane CM, MacCallum RC, et al Stress-related modulation of matrix metalloproteinase expression. *J Neuroimmunol*. 2002;133(1–2):144–150
10. Chiu A, Chon SY, Kimball AB. The response of skin disease to stress: changes in the severity of acne vulgaris as affected by examination stress. *Arch Dermatol*. 2003;139(7):897–900
11. Papadopoulos L, Bor R, Legg C, Hawk JL. Impact of life events on the onset of vitiligo in adults: preliminary evidence for a psychological dimension in aetiology. *Clin Exp Dermatol*. 1998;23(6):243–248
12. Barisic-Drusko V, Rucevic I. Trigger factors in childhood psoriasis and vitiligo. *Coll Antropol*. 2004;28(1):277–285
13. Gulec AT, Tanriverdi N, Duru C, et al The role of psychological factors in alopecia areata and the impact of the disease on the quality of life. *Int J Dermatol*. 2004;43(5):352–356
14. Chaudhary S. Psychosocial stressors in oral lichen planus. *Aust Dental J*. 2004;49(4):192–195
15. Cohen F, Kemeny ME, Kearney KA, et al Persistent stress as a predictor of genital herpes recurrence. *Arch Intern Med*. 1999;159(20):2430–2436
16. Goldberg IA, Brenner S. Pemphigus vulgaris triggered by rifampin and emotional stress. *Skinmed*. 2004;3(5):294
17. Berrino AM, Voltolini S, Fiaschi D, et al Chronic urticaria: importance of a medical-psychological approach. *Allerg Immunol*. 2006;38(5):149–152
18. Naldi L, Peli L, Parazzini F, Carrel CF. Family history of psoriasis, stressful life events, and recent infectious disease are risk factors for a first episode of acute guttate psoriasis: results of a case-control study. *J Am Acad Dermatol*. 2001;44(3):433–438
19. Fortune DG, Richards HL, Griffiths CE, Main CJ. Psychological stress, distress and disability in patients with psoriasis: consensus and variation in the contribution of illness perceptions, coping and alexithymia. *Br J Dermatol*. 2002;41:157–174
20. Fortune DG, Richards HL, Griffiths CE, Main CJ. Psychologic factors in psoriasis: consequences, mechanisms, and interventions. *Dermatol Clin*. 2005;4:681–694
21. Raychaudhuri SP, Farber EM, Raychaudhuri SK. Role of nerve growth factor in RANTES expression by keratinocytes. *Acta Derm Venereol*. 2000;80(4):247–250
22. Nickoloff BJ, Schroeder JM, von den Driesch P, et al Is psoriasis a T-cell disease? *Exp Dermatol*. 2000;9:357–375
23. Farber EM, Nall L. Psoriasis: a stress-related disease. *Cutis*. 1993;51(5):322–326
24. Farber EM, Nickoloff BJ, Recht B, Fraki JE. Stress, symmetry, and psoriasis: possible role of neuropeptides. *J Am Acad Dermatol*. 1986;14(2 Pt 1):305–311
25. Aloe L, Alleva E, Fiore M. Stress and nerve growth factor: findings in animal models and humans. *Pharmacol Biochem Behav*. 2002;73(1):159–166
26. Raychaudhuri SP, Jiang W Y, Farber EM. Psoriatic keratinocytes express high levels of nerve growth factor. *Acta Derm Venereol*. 1998;78(2):84–86
27. Raychaudhuri SP, Jiang W Y, Smoller BR, Farber EM. Nerve growth factor and its receptor system in psoriasis. *Br J Dermatol*. 2000;143(1):198–200
28. Richards HL, Ray DW, Kirby B, et al Response of the hypothalamic-pituitary-adrenal axis to psychological stress in patients with psoriasis. *Br J Dermatol*. 2005;153(6):1114–1120
29. Schmid-Ott GJR, Jaëger B, et al Stress induced endocrine and immunological changes in psoriasis patients and healthy controls. *Psychother Psychosom*. 1998;67:37–42
30. Langan SM, Bourke JF, Silcocks P, Williams HC. An exploratory prospective observational study of environmental factors exacerbating atopic eczema in children. *Br J Dermatol*. 2006;154(5):979–980
31. Faulstich ME, Williamson DA, Duchmann EG, et al Psychophysiological analysis of atopic dermatitis. *J Psychosom Res*. 1985;29(4):415–417
32. Altemus M, Rao B, Dhabhar FS, et al Stress-induced changes in skin barrier function in healthy women. *J Invest Dermatol*. 2001;117(2):309–317
33. Zane L. Psychoneuroendocrinimmunodermatology: pathophysiological mechanisms of stress in cutaneous disease. In: Koo JYM, Lee CS, eds. *Psychocutaneous Medicine*. New York: Marcel Dekker; 2003:65–95
34. Buske-Kirschbaum A, Jobst S, Psych D, et al Attenuated free cortisol response to psychosocial stress in children with atopic dermatitis. *Psychosom Med*. 1997;59(4):419–426
35. Buske-Kirschbaum A, Geiben A, Hollig H, et al Altered responsiveness of the hypothalamus-pituitary-adrenal axis and the sympathetic adrenomedullary system to stress in

patients with atopic dermatitis. *J Clin Endocrinol Metab.* 2002;87(9):4245–4251

36. Rupprecht M, Rupprecht R, Kornhuber J, et al Elevated glucocorticoid receptor concentrations before and after glucocorticoid therapy in peripheral mononuclear leukocytes of patients with atopic dermatitis. *Dermatologica.* 1991;183:100–105

37. Schmid-Ott G, Jaeger B, Meyer S, et al Different expression of cytokine and membrane molecules by circulating lymphocytes on acute mental stress in patients with atopic dermatitis in comparison with healthy controls. *J Allergy Clin Immunol.* 2001;108:455–462

38. Delgado M, Fernandez-Alphonso MS, Fuentes A. Effect of adrenaline and glucocorticoids on monocyte cAMP-specific phospodiesterase (PDE4) in a monocyte cell line. *Arch Dermatol Res.* 2002;294:190–197

39. Theoharides TC, Donelan JM, Papadopoulou N, et al Mast cells as targets of corticotropin-releasing factor and related peptides. *Trends Pharmacol Sci.* 2004;25(11):563–568

40. Papadopoulou N, Kalogeromitros D, Staurianeas NG, et al Corticotropin-releasing hormone receptor-1 and histidine decarboxylase expression in chronic urticaria. *J Invest Dermatol.* 2005;125(5):952–955

41. Biondi M, Zannino LG. Psychological stress, neuroimmunomodulation, and susceptibility to infectious diseases in animals and man: a review. *Psychother Psychosom.* 1997;66 (1):3–26

42. Bailey MT, Engler H, Sheridan JF. Stress induces the translocation of cutaneous and gastrointestinal microflora to secondary lymphoid organs of C57BL/6 mice. *J Neuroimmunol.* 2006;171(1–2):29–37

43. Rojas IG, Padgett DA, Sheridan JF, Marucha PT. Stress-induced susceptibility to bacterial infection during cutaneous wound healing. *Brain Behav Immun.* 2002;16(1):74–84

44. Buske-Kirschbaum A, Geiben A, Wermke C, et al Preliminary evidence for Herpes labialis recurrence following experimentally induced disgust. *Psychother Psychosom.* 2001;70(2):86–91

45. Cohen S, Frank E, Doyle WJ, et al Types of stressors that increase susceptibility to the common cold in healthy adults [see comments]. *Health Psychol.* 1998;17(3):214–223

46. Cohen S, Tyrrell DA, Smith AP. Psychological stress and susceptibility to the common cold [see comments]. *N Engl J Med.* 1991;325(9):606–612

47. VanderPlate C, Kerrick G. Stress reduction treatment of severe recurrent genital herpes virus. *Biofeedback Self Regul.* 1985;10(2):181–188

48. Yang EV, Glaser R. Stress-induced immunomodulation: implications for tumorigenesis. *Brain Behav Immun.* 2003;17 (suppl 1):S37–S40

49. Reiche EM, Nunes SO, Morimoto HK. Stress, depression, the immune system, and cancer. *Lancet Oncol.* 2004;5(10):617–625

50. Reiche EM, Morimoto HK, Nunes SM. Stress and depression-induced immune dysfunction: implications for the development and progression of cancer. *Int Rev Psychiatr.* 2005;17(6):515–527

51. Lillberg K, Verkasalo PK, Kaprio J, et al Stressful life events and risk of breast cancer in 10, 808 women: a cohort study. *Am J Epidemiol.* 2003;157(5):415–423

52. Riley V. Psychoneuroendocrine influences on immunocompetence and neoplasia. *Science.* 1981;212(4499):1100–1109

53. Wu W, Yamaura T, Murakami K, et al Social isolation stress enhanced liver metastasis of murine colon 26–L5 carcinoma cells by suppressing immune responses in mice. *Life Sci.* 2000;66(19):1827–1838

54. Ramirez AJ, Craig TK, Watson JP, et al Stress and relapse of breast cancer [see comments]. *BMJ.* 1989;298(6669):291–293

55. Havlik RJ, Vukasin AP, Ariyan S. The impact of stress on the clinical presentation of melanoma. *Plast Reconstr Surg.* 1992;90(1):57–61; discussion 2–4

56. Reynolds P, Kaplan GA. Social connections and risk for cancer: prospective evidence from the Alameda County Study. *Behav Med.* 1990;16(3):101–110

57. Jacobs JR, Bovasso GB. Early and chronic stress and their relation to breast cancer [In Process Citation]. *Psychol Med.* 2000;30(3):669–678

58. Grossarth-Maticek R, Eysenck HJ, Boyle GJ, et al Interaction of psychosocial and physical risk factors in the causation of mammary cancer, and its prevention through psychological methods of treatment. *J Clin Psychol.* 2000;56(1): 33–50

59. Laudenslager ML, Ryan SM, Drugan RC, et al Coping and immunosuppression: inescapable but not escapable shock suppresses lymphocyte proliferation. *Science.* 1983;221 (4610):568–570

60. Ben-Eliyahu S, Page GG, Yirmiya R, Shakhar G. Evidence that stress and surgical interventions promote tumor development by suppressing natural killer cell activity. *Int J Cancer.* 1999;80(6):880–888

61. Ben-Eliyahu S. The promotion of tumor metastasis by surgery and stress: immunological basis and implications for psychoneuroimmunology. *Brain Behav Immun.* 2003; 17(suppl 1):S27–S36

62. Parker J, Klein SL, McClintock MK, et al Chronic stress accelerates ultraviolet-induced cutaneous carcinogenesis. *J Am Acad Dermatol.* 2004;51(6):919–922

63. Saul AN, Oberyszyn TM, Daugherty C, et al Chronic stress and susceptibility to skin cancer. *J Natl Cancer Inst.* 2005; 97(23):1760–1767

64. Spiegel D, Bloom JR, Kraemer HC, Gottheil E. Effect of psychosocial treatment on survival of patients with metastatic breast cancer [see comments]. *Lancet.* 1989;2(8668):888–891

65. Fawzy FI, Fawzy NW, Hyun CS, et al Malignant melanoma. Effects of an early structured psychiatric intervention, coping, and affective state on recurrence and survival 6 years later. *Arch Gen Psychiatr.* 1993;50(9):681–689

66. Herberman RB, Ortaldo JR. Natural killer cells: their roles in defenses against disease. *Science.* 1981;214:24–30

67. Kiecolt-Glaser JK, Garner W, Speicher C, et al Psychosocial modifiers of immunocompetence in medical students. *Psychosom Med.* 1984;46(1):7–14

68. Glaser R, Rice J, Speicher CE, et al Stress depresses interferon production by leukocytes concomitant with a decrease in natural killer cell activity. *Behav Neurosci.* 1986;100(5):675–678

69. Wu W. Social isolation stress enhanced liver metastasis of murine colon 26–L5 carcinoma cells by suppressing immune responses in mice. *Life Sci.* 2000;66:1827–1838

70. Laudenslager ML. Coping and immunosuppression: inescapable but not escapable shock suppresses lymphocyte proliferation. *Science*. 1983;221:568–570
71. Ernst E. The use of complementary therapies by dermatological patients: a systematic review. *Br J Dermatol*. 2000; 142:857–861
72. Baron SE, Goodwin RG, Nicolau N, et al Use of complementary medicine among outpatients with dermatologic conditions within Yorkshire and South Wales, United Kingdom. *J Am Acad Dermatol*. 2005;52:589–594
73. Nicolaou N, Johnston GA. The use of complementary medicine by patients referred to a contact dermatitis clinic. *Contact Derm*. 2004;51:30–33
74. Augustin M, Zschocke I, Buhrke U. Attitudes and prior experience with respect to alternative medicine among dermatological patients: the Freiburg questionnaire on attitudes to naturopathy (FAN). *Res Complement Med*. 1999;6 (suppl 2): 26–29
75. Chen Yu-Fu, Chang JS. Complementary and alternative medicine use among patients attending a hospital dermatology clinic in Taiwan. *Int J Dermatol*. 2003;42:616–621
76. Simpson EL, Basco M, Hanifin J. Cross-sectional survey of complementary and alternative medicine use in patients with atopic dermatitis. *Am J Contact Derm*. 2003;14:144–147
77. Barnes PM, Powell-Griner E, McFann K, Nahin RL. Complementary and alternative medicine use among adults: United States, 2002. CDC Advance Data Report #343. 2004
78. Rutledge JC, Hyson DA, Garduno D, et al Lifestyle modification program in management of patients with coronary artery disease: the clinical experience in a tertiary care hospital. *J Cardiopulm Rehabil*. 1999;19(4):226–234
79. Luskin FM, Newell KA, Griffith M, et al A review of mind/body therapies in the treatment of musculoskeletal disorders with implications for the elderly. *Altern Ther Health Med*. 2000;6(2):46–56
80. Astin JA, Shapiro SL, Eisenberg DM, et al Mind-body medicine: state of the science, implications for practice. *J Am Board Fam Pract*. 2003;16(2):131–147
81. Mundy EA, DuHamel KN, Montgomery GH. The efficacy of behavioral interventions for cancer treatment-related side effects. *Sem Clin Neuropsychiatr*. 2003;8(4):253–275
82. Irwin MR, Pike JL, Cole JC, et al Effects of a behavioral intervention, Tai Chi Chih, on varicella-zoster virus specific immunity and health functioning in older adults. *Psychosomatic Med*. 2003;65(5):824–830
83. Kiecolt-Glaser JK, Marucha PT, Atkinson C, et al Hypnosis as a modulator of cellular immune dysregulation during acute stress. *J Consult Clin Psychol*. 2001;69(4):674–682
84. yoga.about.com Yoga and Your Health, by Ann Pizer; 2008 Accessed 12.1.08
85. Cancer.gov. Pain control: Support for People with Cancer; 2008 Accessed 25.1.08
86. Deutsch J, Anderson E. *Complementary Therapies for Physical Therapy: A Clinical Decision-Making Approach. Chapter 8: Therapeutic Aspects of Yoga*. St. Louis, MO: Saunders/ Elsevier; 2008
87. Stevensen CJ. Aromatherapy in dermatology. *Clin Dermatol*. 1998;16:689–694
88. Bensouilah J. Psoriasis and aromatherapy. *Int J Aromatherap*. 2003;13:2–8
89. Hosoi J, Tanida M, Tsuchiya T. Mitigation of stress-induced suppression of contact hypersensitivity by odorant inhalation. *Br J Dermatol*. 2001;145:716–719
90. Fujiwara R, Komori T, Noda Y, et al Effects of a long-term inhalation of fragrances on the stress-induced immunosuppression in mice. *Neuroimmunomodulation*. 1998;5(6): 318–322
91. Atsumi T, Tonosaki K. Smelling lavender and rosemary increases free radical scavenging activity and decreases cortisol level in saliva. *Psychiatr Res*. 2007;150:89–96
92. Hay I, Jamieson M, Ormerod AD. Randomized trial of aromatherapy: successful treatment for alopecia areata. *Arch Dermatol*. 1998;134:1349–1352
93. Gaston L, Crombez J, Lassonde M, et al Psychological stress and psoriasis: experimental and prospective correlational studies. *Acta Derm Venereol (Stockh)*. 1991;156:37–43
94. Kabat-Zinn J, Wheeler E, Light T, et al Influence of a mindfulness meditation-based stress reduction intervention on rates of skin clearing in patients with moderate to severe psoriasis undergoing phototherapy (UVB) and photochemotherapy (PUVA). *Psychosomatic Med*. 1998;60:625–632
95. Sarti MG. Biofeedback in dermatology. *Clin Dermatol*. 1998;16:711–714
96. Keinan G, Segal A, Gal U, Brenner S. Stress management for psoriasis patients: the effectiveness of biofeedback and relaxation techniques. *Stress Med*. 1995;11(1):235–241
97. Schenefelt PD. Complementary psychocutaneous therapies in dermatology. *Dermatol Clin*. 2005;23:723–734
98. Bellini MA. Hypnosis in dermatology. *Clin Dermatol*. 1998; 16:725–726
99. Tausk FA, Whitmore E. A pilot study of hypnosis in the treatment of patients with psoriasis. *Psychother Psychosom*. 1998;68:221–225
100. Thomsen RJ. Spirituality in medical practice. *Arch Derm*. 1998;134:1443–1446
101. Sollner W, Zingg-Schir M, Rumpold G, Fritsch P. Attitude toward alternative therapy, compliance with standard treatment, and need for emotional support in patients with melanoma. *Arch Derm*. 1997;133:316–321
102. Branzzini B, Ghersetich I, Hercogava J, Lotti T. The neuro-immuno-cutaneous-endocrine network: relationship between mind and skin. *Dermatol Ther*. 2003;16:123–131
103. Harth W, Gieler U, Kusnir D, Tausk FA. *Clinical Management of Psychodermatology*. Heidelberg: Springer; 2009

Robert A. Norman and Max J. Rappaport

It is well-known that costs for medical problems associated with smoking, obesity, malnutrition, and sun damage are very high, making it extremely important to push the notion of prevention in all of these cases. Between 1995 and 1999, it has been estimated that the United States spent $157 billion in healthcare costs.[1] The costs associated with medical costs in the United States attributed to inactivity alone are around $75 billion.[2] Many medical issues are preventable, which an uninformed person may not realize. But information on the risks of smoking, obesity, or tanning is well-documented and readily available. Still today there are around 1.25 billion smokers who will die an average of 7 years earlier than their nonsmoking counterparts.[3] About 30% of people worldwide are considered to obese and the numbers have been increasing dramatically ever since the 1980s.[4,5] Every year according to the World Health Organization (WHO),[6] sun damage causes 60,000 premature deaths and the loss of 1.5 million disability-adjusted life years (DALYs); in addition almost 30 million Americans tan indoors every year.[7] Health risks associated with these three high – risk factors have become common knowledge in many countries. Yet doctors see patients seeking healthcare related to damage done by one or more of these risks time and time again. The most difficult and expensive approach will always be to treat the complications related to a risky behavior after an accumulation of damage, thus – as with anything else in life – preventing a problem before it occurs is always the best option.

All three of these risky behaviors are preventable. Positive behavioral changes, even after damage, can be extremely beneficial to a person's future health.

2.1 Smoking

The dangers of smoking cigarettes have become well-known; though the damage to the skin has been less studied. The smoke released from burning cigarettes at temperatures of 830–900°C contains some 5,000 chemicals. Many of these are hydrophobic agents that can diffuse through many cell membranes, reaching to the far ends of the body's precious organs, including the skin.[3,8] Many of the dangerous chemicals are in the form of free radicals and oxidants, which can cause the malfunction of many biological functions and create cell damage. Smoking has been shown to increase many symptoms associated with aging: altered hormone production, reduced fertility, cancer, cardiovascular and respiratory disease, and diseases of the lung, esophagus, pharynx, larynx, stomach, pancreas, bladder, uterine, cervix, and skin.[3,8–10]

Smoking causes premature aging of the skin by affecting the color, tone, and wrinkling. Smoking can also increase the risk for developing psoriasis, melanoma, squamous cell carcinomas on lips and oral mucosa, acne, and hair loss. Smoking also causes poor wound healing due to reduction of oxygen and nutrients to the skin.[9,11–14] Many of the mechanisms that can explain these findings are complex and inexact. Premature skin aging may be caused in part by the same mechanisms which seem to cause the entire body's aging process.[15] The premature death of smokers follows similar old-age-related illnesses of non-smokers such as osteoporosis, cancers, macular degeneration,

R.A. Norman (✉)
Nova Southeastern University,
Ft. Lauderdale, FL, USA and
Private Practice, Tampa,
FL, USA
e-mail: skindrrob@aol.com

and cardiovascular diseases.[12] The acceleration of aging in smokers may be caused in part by actual damage to the body or from destruction of chemicals needed to prevent aging in the body by causing molecular malfunctioning, leading to an increase in tumor development and a reduction in wound healing.[3] Another theory on the causation of premature wrinkling of the skin may be increased elastosis in the skin. It has been found that the amount of wrinkling is directly related with the amount and duration of cigarettes smoked. The mechanism by which wrinkling occurs on the skin may be the same as the mechanism by which collagen and elastin in the lungs are damaged. Lastly, there is an idea that the skin damage is caused by extended exposure to intense heat while smoking.[12] Smoking also affects the levels of antioxidants in the body, accounting for premature aging. Many of the chemicals in the cigarette smoke cause damage that has been shown to decrease cutaneous blood flow and immune responses in the blood and decrease the level of vitamin C, vitamin E, circulating levels of nitrous oxide, and plasma concentrations, while increasing lipid peroxidation.[8]

Health damage and premature deaths caused by smoking are in a large part preventable. An emphasis on preventing new smokers is important because quitting can be a difficult process. Every year almost 15 million smokers attempt to quit smoking in the United States, with around one million in specific cessation programs.[13] This very small proportion of the actual smokers shows how difficult quitting can be. While people hear from everyone around them, including the media, that smoking is bad for their health, a healthcare provider must always push further intervention. Talking to parents of pediatric patients and directly to pediatric patients as early as possible is the primary role of the physician. Increasing education in schools about the dangers of smoking can also be a powerful tool to reduce new smoking behavior. It has been shown that health education programs using negative images to discourage smoking is more effective than positive images.[16] Actual, real-life, positive role modeling by older students, parents, and teachers may be just as effective. While young smokers imagine the typical smoker as smart, good-looking, and considerate, nonsmokers perceive smokers as dull, childish, and confused. Reinforcement of the nonsmokers'

beliefs is important by positive role modeling.[16] For youths who have already begun smoking, knowledge that smoking may increase the rate of facial aging may increase their likeliness of quitting.[13] Informing young smokers of the positive health benefits of quitting may be a powerful tool. It is known, for example, that the risk of psoriasis decreases with every year of smoking cessation and becomes insignificant 20 years after a smoker has quit.[13]

2.2 Obesity and Nutrition

Obesity is another preventable disorder that, if gone untreated, can lead to a number of medical complications including orthopedic and metabolic problems, disrupted sleep, weakened immune system, impaired mobility, increased blood pressure, and hypertension. Psychosocial consequences include low self-esteem and depression. Long-term consequences include cardiovascular disease, insulin resistance, type 2 diabetes, hyperlipidemia, gall bladder disease, osteoarthritis, and certain cancers. When looking at prevention, it is important to note that obese children tend to grow into obese adults.[4]

Skin complications related to obesity include[5,17,18]:

- Acanthosis nigricans
- Acrochordons
- Keratosis pilaris
- Hyperandrogenism and hirsutism
- Striae distensae
- Adiposis dolorosa and fat redistribution
- Lymphedema
- Chronic venous insufficiency
- Plantar hyperkeratosis
- Cellulitis
- Hidradenitis suppurativa
- Psoriasis
- Insulin resistance syndrome
- Tophaceous gout
- Changes in cutaneous sensation and temperature regulation
- Foot pain
- Candidiasis
- Intertrigo

- Candida folliculosis
- Erythrasma
- Tinea cruris
- Folliculitis
- Necrotizing fasciitis
- Gas gangrene
- Leg ulcerations
- Plantar hyperkeratosis

Skin disorders attributed to malnutrition include scurvy, pellagra, ariboflavinosis, vitamin A deficiency, phrynoderma, and kwashiorkor.[19,20] Treatment of obese patients can also lead to a number of complications including difficulty in treating wounds and abnormal medicine dosages.[5]

Obesity prevention and nutritional education to the youth must be a powerful tool in the fight to prevent more obese adults. There are a number of factors that may be affecting the increased prevalence in obesity both in adults and in children. The list includes the individual's genetic makeup including psychological tendencies; the individual family's eating habits and amount of active behaviors while at school, school food, availability of vending machines, and cheap and readily available high-calorie, low-nutrition foods including fast foods. While many factors such as genetics and societal may not be readily changed, prevention will always be easier than treatment.

Treating at-risk overweight kids before they become obese is extremely important. Care must be taken in school-based obesity prevention programs to prevent stigmatizing overweight children or pushing already underweight children further in that dangerous direction. Four prevention programs must promote exercise, how to eat healthily, and the dangers associated with becoming obese. The most effective prevention plans must be effective, sustainable, and not harm the participants. Extreme low-calorie diets (<700 daily calories) with a lack of fruits, vegetables, fish, and eggs can lead to a deficiency in many essential vitamins and cause malnutrition disorders, such as phrynoderma, usually found in undeveloped nations. If detected early, diets rich in the missing vitamins and nutrients can be implemented to prevent these disorders.[20] Positive role modeling and education must be used by all those who teach or influence children from the earliest age possible, of the dangers and risks of not taking care of their bodies.

2.3 Sun Damage

Many societies today value the appearance of a dark, rich tan, causing many people to expose themselves to high levels of ultraviolet radiation (UVR) without the necessary and available protection to prevent illnesses associated with sun damage. Many factors affect the level of UVR a person can receive yearly, from distal factors such as ozone levels, cloud cover, latitude, season, and lower atmospheric pollution, to proximal factors such as sun-seeking, sun-protecting behaviors, genetic skin pigmentation, and cultural dress and behaviors.[6] UVR damage can suppress cell-mediated immunity in the body, have an adverse affect on the eyes and skin, and increase the risk of cancer. Absence of UVR can produce an insufficiency of vitamin D, increasing the risk of other complications including rickets, osteomalacia, osteoporosis, and tuberculosis.[21]

The skin is especially susceptible to damage from the sun; it is the first organ of the body to come in contact with UVR rays and covers the entire surface of the body. Specific damage to the skin caused by sun damage include malignant melanoma, cancer of the lip, squamous cell carcinoma, basal cell carcinoma, sunburn, photo-aging (wrinkles), psoriasis, and other photodermatoses such as solar urticaria, photoallergic contact dermatitis, actinic prurigo, polymorphic light eruption, and hydroa vacciniforme.[21]

Any skin damage caused by the sun is almost entirely preventable. For proper protection sunscreen with reapplications is necessary; wearing hats and long-sleeve shirts when in the sun is also recommended. Be aware of your risk category; people with lighter skin tend to burn more easily. People who spend their work days out-of-doors should be aware of the risks and take similar precautions.

A general risk that should be addressed by the physician is the fact that intentional sun damage to gain a tan, even if using sunscreen, is a risk for all the same skin damages caused by sun damage without sunscreen. Knowledge on the damages caused by the sun is well-known and yet ignored by too many of today's youth and adults.

2.4 Synergy of Risk and Integrating Prevention

It is clear that smoking, exposure to UVR rays, obesity, and poor nutrition can lead to a number or dermatological issues that are entirely preventable. It has been noted that persons who participate in one type of risky behavior are more likely to participate in others. Therefore, it is necessary to consider that a combination of risk factors may be synergistic in nature, thus accelerating damage by just one risk factor. When looking at prevention, education in all of these risk factors must be addressed in part and as a whole. Positive role modeling by older peers, teachers, parents, and even physicians is extremely important in the battle of prevention. It has been noted that the more ambiguous a prevention plan is and the larger the number of possible options it offers, the more it is perceived with skepticism about its effectiveness and the more it is met with inaction.[22]

Another tool in fighting the three risks simultaneously is directing education at those in the process of smoking cessation, as persons trying to change one aspect of their life may be more inclined to change other aspects of their life at the same time.[23] Finally, it is clear that action taken must be aimed at the younger populations to further educate persons on the risks associated with risky behaviors and the ease of preventing the harmful and deadly effects of smoking, malnutrition, obesity, and sun damage.

References

1. World Health Organization. World No Tobacco Day 2004. Tobacco and Poverty: A Vicious Circle. http://www.emro.who.int/tfi/wntd2004/Kit-Part1.htm; 2008 Accessed 29.12.08
2. World Health Organization. Physical Activity. http://www.who.int/dietphysicalactivity/publications/facts/pa/en/; 2008 Accessed 29.12.08
3. Bernhard D, Moser C, Aleksandar Backovic A, Wick G. Cigarette smoke – an aging accelerator? Exp Gerontol. 2007; 42:160–165
4. Doak CM, Visscher TLS, Renders CM, Seidell JC. The prevention of overweight and obesity in children and adolescents: a review of interventions and programmes. Obes Rev. 2006;7:111–136
5. Scheinfeld NS. Obesity and dermatology. Clin Dermatol. 2004;22:303–309
6. Lucas R, Prüss-Üstün A, World Health Organization, et al Solar ultraviolet eadiation: global burden of disease from solar ultraviolet radiation. Environmental Burden of Disease Series, No. 13. http://www.who.int/uv/publications/solar-adgbd/en/index.html; 2008 Accessed 28.12.08
7. Jung K, Seifert M, Herrling T, Fuchs J. UV-generated free radicals (FR) in the skin: their prevention by sunscreens and their induction by self-tanning agents. Spectrochim Acta Part A Mol Biomol Spectrosc. 2008;69(5):1423–1428. Epub 2007
8. Nicita-Mauro V, Lo Balbo C, Mento A, et al Smoking, aging and the centenarians. Exp Gerontol. 2008;43(2):95–101
9. Merimsky O, Inbar M. Cigarette smoking and skin cancer. Clin Dermatol. 1998;16:585–588
10. Shulman A, Wolf R. Cigarette smoking, hormonal changes, and the skin. Clin Dermatol. 1998;16:595–598
11. Morita A. Tobacco smoke causes premature skin aging. J Dermatol Sci. 2007;48:169–175
12. Boyd AS, Stasko T, Lloyd E, et al Cigarette smoking– associated elastotic changes in the skin. J Am Acad Dermatol. 1999;41:23–26
13. Setty AR, Curhan G, Choi HK. Smoking and the risk of psoriasis in women: Nurses' Health Study II. Am J Med. 2007; 120:953–959
14. Odenbro A, Gillgren P, Bellocco R, et al The risk for cutaneous malignant melanoma, melanoma in situ and intraocular malignant melanoma in relation to tobacco use and body mass index. Br J Dermatol. 2007;156:99–105
15. Demierre MF, Brooks D, Koh HK, Geller AC. Public knowledge, awareness, and perceptions of the association between skin aging and smoking. J Am Acad Dermatol. 1999; 41(1): 27–30
16. Piko BF, Bak J, Gibbons FX. Prototype perception and smoking: are negative or positive social images more important in adolescence? Addict Behav. 2007;32:1728–1732
17. Hidalgo LG. Dermatological complications of obesity. Am J Clin Dermatol. 2002;3(7):497–506
18. Yosipovitch G, DeVore A, Dawn A. Obesity and the skin: skin physiology and skin manifestations of obesity. J Am Acad Dermatol. 2007;56:901–916
19. Lee B Y, Hogan DJ, Ursine S, et al Personal observation of skin disorders in malnutrition. Clin Dermatol. 2006;24: 222–227
20. Di Stefani AD, Orlandi A, Chimenti S, Bianchi L. Phrynoderma: a cutaneous sign of an inadequate diet. CMAJ. 2007;177(8):855–856
21. World Health Organization: WHO Annexes: Annex 1. www.who.int/entity/uv/health/solaruvradann1.pdf; 2008 Accessed 28.12.08
22. Han PKJ, Moscr RP, Klein WMP. Perceived ambiguity about cancer prevention recommendations: associations with cancer-related perceptions and behaviours in a U.S. population survey. Health Expect. 2007;10:321–336
23. Simmons VN, Vidrine JI, Brandon TH. Smoking cessation counseling as a teachable moment for skin cancer prevention: pilot studies. Am J Health Behav. 2008;32(2):137–145

Raising Awareness on the Health Literacy Epidemic

3

Michelle C. Duhaney

Low health literacy is common in the United States of the twenty-first century. The ability to process and understand basic health information and function appropriately in today's healthcare environment requires basic reading and mathematical skills.[1,2] These basic skills are often taken for granted by patients with adequate health literacy. It is likely that most physicians will encounter on a daily basis patients who cannot read or spell, which is a barrier to accurate medical diagnosis and optimal treatment.[3]

The magnitude of the association between inadequate health literacy and mortality has captured the attention of many. The nature of this problem is complex and effectively addressing it is important to America's well-being.[4] In a study of elderly patients enrolling in a Medicare-managed care plan, inadequate health literacy independently predicted all-cause mortality and death due to cardiovascular events. This study concluded that the crude mortality rate for patients with inadequate health literacy was relatively high at 39.4%.[5] In an era that has seen breakthrough drug regimens and life-saving treatments the effect of low health literacy on the mortality rate is alarming.[2,5]

Health literacy is therefore gaining momentum among researchers. Research over the last 15 years has attempted to assess the nature and scope of health literacy and the impact that low health literacy has on the delivery of quality healthcare in the United States[3,4] Several studies have shown that patients with inadequate health literacy have decreased knowledge and understanding about diseases, especially chronic diseases such as diabetes and hypertension.[5,6] Patients with inadequate health literacy also have decreased medication adherence, increased involvement in risky health behaviors, and a poor understanding of preventive health measures.[6,7]

Low health literacy impacts more than the mortality rate; patients with inadequate health literacy have increased rates of hospitalization. If not appropriately addressed, America's healthcare costs will continue to rise.[6]

Many researchers have documented the relationship between health literacy of adults in the United States and adverse health outcomes. A limited number of studies have been done, however, to assess the link between parental/caregiver health literacy and the health outcome of our nation's children.[5] In the few studies that have been documented, low parental health literacy has been linked to behaviors that negatively impact a child's health.[5] A patient's level of education, age, race, ethnicity, and culture also impact the outcome of healthcare, contribute to patient compliance, and even affect healthcare costs.[1,8] It is not surprising, therefore, that by improving literacy, health outcomes will also improve.

Many cognitive assessment tools are now available to measure health literacy. These tools assess a patient's recognition of medical terms and ability to interpret written health materials.[1] Since approximately 90 million adults have fair-to-poor literacy and 21–23% of adults read at the lowest reading level, other interventions such as educational videotapes or DVDs and color-coded medication schedules may improve the delivery of healthcare.[1,9] America has realized that quality healthcare relies on effective communication between patients and involving members of the healthcare team. Although attempts have been made to increase health literacy and in turn improve patients'

M.C. Duhaney
Department of Family Medicine,
Broward General Medical Centre,
Fort Lauderdale, FL, USA
e-mail: doctorduhaney@gmail.com

understanding through effective communication, the scope is not broad enough and certainly the pace is not fast enough to make the progress that is necessary.[4, 10] Awareness of this epidemic must be further increased and more research should be done.[11]

3.1 Introduction

Health literacy has been defined "as the degree to which individuals have the capacity to obtain, process and understand basic health information and services needed to make appropriate health decisions."[12] The American Medical Association (AMA) expanded on the definition and defined health literacy "as a constellation of skills" which includes the ability to do basic reading and perform basic numerical tasks.[1] A patient's inability to perform these basic tasks acts as a barrier to accurate medical diagnosis and optimal treatment. This inadequacy of health literacy contributes to a weak healthcare system in the United States. Patients become noncompliant, chronic diseases become more difficult to control, and healthcare costs continue to rise.[1] A significant proportion of adults in the United States are impacted by this epidemic. According to a report from the Institute of Medicine (IOM), almost 50% of Americans have difficulty understanding basic printed health information.[1, 7] The 2003 national assessment of adult literacy (NAAL) revealed that approximately 90 million American adults have fair-to-poor literacy.[1, 12] Effective patient–physician communication is therefore the key element to accurate medical diagnosis and optimal treatment. It is recommended that physicians elicit patient comprehension of disease processes.[13] Effective communication will lead to improved patient satisfaction and medication adherence and subsequently improved health outcome.[11, 13, 14] Physicians also need to be cognizant that health literacy is compounded by a patient's age, race and ethnicity, culture, language spoken, and historical experiences with racial and ethnic disparities that have led to mistrust of the healthcare system.[1, 15]

3.2 Epidemiology

In today's society, the patients with the greatest healthcare needs may have the least ability to perform basic reading and mathematical tasks.[11] A recent government study estimated that over 89 million American adults have limited health literacy.[1] A systematic review estimated that 21–23% of adults read at the lowest reading level which is approximately fifth grade or lower.[1] Inadequate health literacy in America is surprisingly common. A 2003 survey categorized US health literacy rates into four groups: proficient (11%), intermediate (53%), basic (22%), and below basic (14%).[16] Health literacy becomes more complicated in elderly patients and in patients whose primary language is not English. Elderly patients may have a limited ability to read information pertinent to their health because of declining cognitive and sensory function.[1, 17] In fact, the majority of patients older than 60 years have inadequate literacy.[1] The ability to read and comprehend prescription bottles, appointment slips, and other essential health-related materials is decreased in the elderly.[1, 15] Approximately 80% of the elderly in the United States have a limited ability in filling out forms, such as those requested in physician waiting rooms.[1] A survey of patients at two US public hospitals revealed that 35% of English-speaking patients and 62% of Spanish-speaking patients had fair-to-poor health literacy.[1, 9] A majority of these patients may avoid seeking medical attention because they are in denial or because they are embarrassed.[1] Limited health literacy has been linked to delayed medical diagnosis.[6, 18] Once a diagnosis is made, physicians may encounter patients who have a difficulty understanding their medical condition and the need for using preventive health measures.[6, 18] Adherence to medical instructions and self-management skills may also become problematic.[6]

Not only is there an association between low health literacy and morbidity, but low health literacy has been linked to an increase in the mortality rate. A 5-year prospective study of 2,500 adults with the average age of 75.6 was analyzed. After adjusting for demographic and socioeconomic status (SES), comorbid conditions and patient-health-related behaviors, there was a two-fold increase in the mortality rate.[18] In another prospective study, the crude mortality rate for patients with inadequate health literacy was 39.4%. The rates for the participants with marginal and adequate health literacy were 28.7 and 18.9% respectively.[5]

The NAAL survey estimated that 14% of adults in the United States have below basic level of *prose literacy*, the ability to use "printed and written information to function in society, to achieve one's goals, and to develop one's knowledge and potential."[9] *Document literacy* is the ability to read and comprehend documents such as drug or food labels.[9] Twelve percent of adult patients are estimated to have below basic document literacy.[9] Many patients are unable to understand prescription labels. Although 71% with inadequate health literacy correctly said "Take two tablets by mouth twice daily," only 35% could demonstrate this instruction in a study done to assess patient comprehension.[19] Another report found that 24–58% of patients did not understand directions to take a medication on an empty stomach.[19] The NAAL survey also showed that 22% of adults are estimated to have below basic *quantitative literacy*. Quantitative literacy is defined as the ability to perform quantitative or mathematical tasks. Patients with inadequate quantitative literacy may be able to add up all the numbers on a bank slip, but they cannot, for example, compare ticket prices for some events.[9] The elderly are more likely to have chronic and multiple medical comorbid conditions. These patients may have a difficult time with health literacy because of decreased sensory and cognitive function and as a result may have a difficult time controlling their chronic and comorbid conditions.[1,17] On the basis of NAAL, it was analyzed that the patients over the age of 64 with below basic prose literacy, basic document literacy, and basic quantitative literacy accounted for 23, 27, and 34% respectively.[9]

3.3 Health Literacy Assessment Tools

During the past decade, the magnitude of the health literacy epidemic in America and the effect it has had on health outcome and mortality has received considerable attention. Patients with inadequate health literacy have a complex array of difficulties which influence diagnosis and disease management.[6,11] It remains unclear whether screening patients for health literacy improves health outcome. A common mistake is to rely on patients' own assessment of their level of health literacy. The majority of patients who have inadequate health literacy will say that they know more than they really do and overstate their reading competence.[1] Patients with low literacy often are too embarrassed to admit that they do not understand and therefore refuse to ask their physician to explain or repeat relevant information regarding their health.[1] Many have told no one about their handicap including their spouses and family members. Although the evidence is insufficient to conclude that screening improves patient–physician

communication and subsequently morbidity and mortality, many types of standardized literacy assessment tools are now available.[1,5] They measure the health literacy and assess a patient's recognition of healthcare terms. They also assess a patient's ability to interpret written health materials.[1] The rapid estimate of adult literacy in medicine (REALM) and test of functional health literacy in adults (TOFHLA) were developed specifically to measure patients' health literacy.[7] Although both the REALM and TOFHLA are valid and easily administered, the REALM is the most commonly used tool.[7] Since its introduction in 1991 the REALM has been identified as the quickest of the two, taking less than 5 min to complete and can easily be administered by a nurse or other members of the medical staff.[1] The REALM is a word recognition test. It is comprised of 66 medical terms that are arranged in order of increasing complexity.[7] During the administration of this test patients are asked to read down the list and pronounce as many words as they can. The examiner uses standard dictionary pronunciation as the scoring standard and assigns a score based on the number of words pronounced correctly.[7] One point is given for each word that is correctly pronounced. Scores therefore vary from 0 to 66. A score of 0 indicates that none of the words were pronounced correctly and a score of 66 indicates that all the words were pronounced correctly.[7] The scores are then matched to a grade equivalent. A score of 0–18 would be equivalent to third grade or less, 19–44 would be equivalent to fourth to sixth grade, 45–60 would be equivalent to seventh to eighth grade and 61–66 would be equivalent to high school.[1,7] The TOFHLA is also available for use by healthcare professionals and is available in both Spanish and English. Although the TOFHLA provides a more thorough assessment of a patient's ability to comprehend, it is less practical for today's use and it is more time-consuming.[1] It takes approximately 22 min to administer.[7] There is a short form of TOFHLA called the S-TOFHLA that takes approximately 7 min.[7]

In a well-written report, the validity of a new and rapid literacy assessment instrument was discussed. The newest vital sign (NVS) was introduced in 2005 with the intention of addressing the speed and accuracy of health literacy assessment.[12] NVS is now available in both English and Spanish and uses the TOFHLA as the reference standard.[20] NVS was developed from a series of scenarios that were created by a panel of health literacy experts. The candidate scenarios included instructions from a prescription for headache medicine, a consent form for coronary angiography, instructions for self-care and management of heart failure, an ice cream nutrition label, and instructions for an asthma medication that included a tapering steroid dose.[12] Patients were asked to read these health-related scenarios and then demonstrate their ability to use the information by answering certain questions about each scenario.[20] Since one has to be able to do basic reading and perform basic mathematical tasks in order to survive in today's healthcare environment, some of the scenarios did involve both reading and mathematical concepts.[1,12,20] The scenario that best determined the literacy level was the one with the ice cream nutrition label.[12] The average completion time for the English version was 2.9 min. The Spanish version took on average more time to complete.[12] In detecting marginal health literacy, NVS may be more sensitive than TOFHLA. The specificity of NVS is similar to or better than other screening tools such as the widely used CAGE questionnaires to detect alcohol abuse and the screening methods to detect arthritis.[20] Like REALM and TOFHLA, NVS has its limitations. The Spanish version was not as good as the English version.[20] The primary care practices that were involved in the study did not fully represent all primary care practices. They were selected because they had a high percentage of Spanish-speaking patients. Among these Spanish-speaking patients the percentage of males was relatively small.[20] Despite these limitations the NVS has advantages over the REALM and TOFHLA. In the future, studies should examine the validity of NVS in both primary and nonprimary care setting and whether raising a physician's awareness to the issue of health literacy results in better health outcome.[20]

During the last 15 years, research has shown that patients with inadequate health literacy often have a poorer understanding of their medical diagnosis and are less likely to utilize disease management techniques. These patients tend to underuse health promoting and disease prevention programs and often engage themselves in risky health behaviors.[7] The number of patients that are affected is alarming. On the basis of these findings, more research should concentrate on improving screening methods. Physicians should also pay special attention to informal behavioral cues that may help detect low health literacy. Patients with inadequate health literacy often attempt to identify their medications by looking at the pill instead of the medication

label. Other behavioral cues include frequent misspelling or turning in incomplete medical forms.[12] Making excuses and mimicking others may also be signs suggestive of inadequate health literacy.[1]

3.4 The Nature of This Epidemic

The magnitude and the consequence of low health literacy are of concern to many, especially when one considers the effect it has had on morbidity and mortality. Many researchers describe low literacy as a silent epidemic.[9] The problems are numerous and complex and for that reason health literacy has been receiving considerable attention. Patients with inadequate health literacy have a difficult time using the healthcare system. These patients may refuse to keep doctor's appointments because they may not be able to register for health insurance or even follow simple driving directions. Once these patients arrive at the office they may not be able to complete medical forms because they cannot read or follow simple instructions and once that appointment is over they may not know when to follow up.[1] Physicians should be alert for this problem because most patients are too embarrassed to admit that they have a literacy issue. Patients with inadequate health literacy are less likely to participate in health promotion and disease prevention programs. They have a poor understanding of disease-preventive measures such as pap smears, mammography, and colonoscopy. Not only do these patients have less basic health knowledge and worse self-management skills, but they are more likely to be hospitalized.[1,6] Even after adjusting for other factors associated with increased risk for hospitalization, studies conclude that patients with inadequate health literacy are more likely to be hospitalized.[12] Patients with inadequate health literacy have 29–52% higher hospitalization rates.[5] One study showed that adult males with inadequate health literacy would commonly present with advanced stage prostate cancer. It was suggested that those with inadequate health literacy delayed seeking medical attention and presented in the very late stages of the disease.[12] Other diseases like diabetes and hypertension require a patient to be health literate in order to be adequately controlled. Diabetes and hypertension are chronic diseases that require the patient to be educated to avoid adverse health outcomes.[14] Patients with hypertension may need to understand how to take multiple medications. The intricacies involved with self-management of diabetes often get ignored in a patient with inadequate health literacy. Patients with inadequate reading and mathematical skills often have a difficult time monitoring home glucose levels and administering insulin.[14] In an observational study of 408 patients with type 2 diabetes, inadequate literacy was associated with poor glycemic control and an increase in the rate of diabetic retinopathy.[21] In another study of over 500 patients hospitalized for diabetes, only 50% of patients with inadequate literacy knew the symptoms of hypoglycemia compared to 94% with adequate literacy.[14] Ninety-two percent of patients with hypertension who had adequate literacy knew that a blood pressure reading of 160/100 mmHg was high while only 55% of patients with low health literacy were able to evaluate this reading.[14]

3.5 Education and Health Literacy

A patient's level of education plays a vital role in their understanding that lifestyle and behavioral modifications are required when managing diseases. Especially when managing diabetes and hypertension, health literacy must be up to par to achieve adequate control and to prevent adverse outcomes such as death.[14] Most health-related materials are written at the tenth grade level or higher. The majority of adults have a difficult time comprehending these health-related materials since most adults read between the eighth and ninth grade level.[1] Patients with poor reading and poor mathematical skills may have a difficult time reading food labels and calculating calories. Health literacy is thus associated with diet and medication adherence. In a report of 2,659 predominantly poor patients at two public hospitals, up to 58% of patients did not understand the direction to take a medication on an empty stomach.[14] Proper medication administration is crucial to adequate disease management. Physicians need to elicit their patients' understanding. Evidence clearly links patient–physician communication to patient adherence and health outcome. Patients in general recall or comprehend as little as half of what physicians convey.[13] This is even lower in a patient with inadequate literacy. In a study that used direct

observation to measure the extent to which primary care physicians assess patient recall and comprehension during diabetic patient encounters, it was found that these physicians rarely assessed recall or comprehension of new concepts.[13] This reflects a missed opportunity to improve and enhance patient compliance and ultimately improve disease management.[13] There is clear evidence that improving a patient's comprehension of a disease improves medication adherence and disease outcome. Ensuring recall and comprehension becomes especially important in our diabetic and hypertensive patients since they must cope with the complex nature of their disease and the intricacies of self-management.[13]

3.6 Age and Health Literacy

The impact of age on clinical care is important. As age increases, so do the deficits in literacy.[1] Elderly patients may have a difficult time reading and comprehending information regarding their health because of an increased time since formal education. Decreased cognitive and sensory function also compounds this problem of health literacy. The majority of patients older than 60 years have low health literacy. Eighty percent have a difficult time filling out forms such as insurance forms and the ones they have to complete in physician waiting rooms.[1] To determine the prevalence of low functional health literacy among Medicare enrollees, a cross-sectional survey of new enrollees in health plans of a national managed care organization was done.[6,17] After adjusting for years of school completed and cognitive impairment, a patient's reading ability was seen to decline with age.[17] Approximately 30% of English-speaking patients and 50% of Spanish-speaking patients had low or marginal health literacy.[17] The study concluded that elderly managed care enrollees may not be able to function appropriately in a healthcare setting. Low health literacy may impair their understanding and thus limit their ability to care for themselves and their medical problems.[17] Higher total medical and emergency costs are associated with low health literacy in the elderly. Patients tend to avoid outpatient doctors' offices because they are embarrassed about their inability to fill out paperwork. They may find emergency rooms easier to use because information is taken and forms filled out by others.[9]

Elderly patients with low health literacy and high prevalence of chronic conditions may have increased levels of depression.[22] Investigators also sought to determine whether older adults with inadequate health literacy were more likely to report depressive symptoms.[22] Overall, 13% of the respondents were classified as being depressed.[22] Although some patients with inadequate health literacy are unaware of their handicap; others feel significant shame and decreased worth.[1,22] One study found that among those patients who admitted that they had a reading problem, the majority did not disclose this information to their spouse or family[22]; 19% of subjects had never even disclosed their inability to read to their healthcare provider.[22] Such embarrassment may lead to social isolation. It is possible that these feelings of embarrassment and shame could lead to a higher prevalence of depression. In fact, individuals in the study who had less social support had significantly higher odds of being depressed.[22] Data generally suggest that the higher the level of education a person attains the fewer depressed symptoms they will have. Some studies propose that this may be due to a greater financial success, improved lifestyle behaviors, and improved problem-solving capacity.[22] The investigators also sought to determine whether the potential relationship between health literacy and depression may be mediated by health status. Some literature suggests that there is a strong predictive power of health status on depression.[22] Especially among the elderly, there may be higher rates of depression because of low health literacy coupled with a high prevalence of chronic conditions.[22] Even after controlling for other factors, it was found that individuals who were inactive and exercised less than twice a week were twice as likely to have symptoms of depression.[22] In the cross-sectional survey, patients with low health literacy were more likely to report that they were depressed than those patients with adequate health literacy. This was mostly explained by their worse health status. This relationship between depression and poor health status suggests the need to research ways to improve patients' health.

Patients may need to be referred for social support to help with their depression and exercise programs to increase exercise tolerance and compliance.[22]

3.7 Parental Health Literacy and Pediatric Health

Health literacy is now gaining momentum among researchers. Many studies have been done to assess the relationship between adult health literacy and health outcomes. A limited number of studies have been done to evaluate the association between parental literacy and a child's health outcome. In the few studies that have been done, low parental health literacy has been linked to behaviors that have a negative impact on children's health.[12] The REALM was utilized in a study of 600 pregnant women. After controlling for age, race, marital status, living with a smoker, and current smoking status, the study concluded that pregnant women with inadequate health literacy had significantly less knowledge about the negative effects that smoking had on their babies' health.[12] In fact, 66% of the pregnant women with at least a ninth grade level of education were more concerned about the effects of smoking and their babies' health as compared to only 37% of women who had a third grade level of education or lower.[12] The issue of not initiating breastfeeding and how this may affect a baby's health were also studied. A study done by Kaufman and coworkers on primarily low SES mothers showed that those women with at least a ninth grade education were more likely to breastfeed for at least 2 months. This was estimated to be 54% as compared to 23% of parents with a seventh or eighth grade level of education.[12] All parents are required to receive information on childhood immunization. One study found that this information is written above the tenth grade level of reading. In fact, a study of documents available through the American Academy of Pediatrics found that the reading levels of asthma management plans ranged from eighth grade to twelfth grade.[12] Most adults in the United States read at the eighth grade level and below.[1] One study assessed asthma care measures in children who presented for care in an outpatient clinic and found that children of parents with low health literacy were more likely to have emergency department visits and had more hospitalizations.[12] Screening for parents/caregivers is not easy. Most physicians do not screen parents due to time constraints and they may also lack the knowledge on how to intervene when they discover that a parent has inadequate health literacy.[12]

3.8 Childhood and Adolescent Health Literacy

There may be a link between child and adolescent health literacy and their own health outcome. Only a limited number of studies have been done to assess this possible link.[12] One study was done on 3,000 students in Australia that found an association between adolescent literacy level and substance use, namely tobacco.[12] The same study concluded that there is a link between the health literacy of adolescent boys and alcohol misuse.[12] A study done of over 350 US children concluded that there is a link between low literacy and carrying weapons and participating in fights at school.[12] Recently a study was done to assess the link between child health literacy, parent health literacy and childhood obesity. Adjustments were made for the children's age, gender, insurance, eating-self efficacy, exercise self efficacy, exercise activity, grade in school and reported reading level and the parents' primary language spoken at home and body mass index.[12] After adjusting these confounders it was found that low child health literacy as opposed to low parent health literacy had an association with body mass index Z-scores.[12] Although research is limited, some studies have concluded that a child's health is impacted not only by parental/care-giver health literacy but also by the health literacy of the child. It is unclear whether screening children and adolescent for health literacy is necessary. In December 2006, a screening tool called the REALM-Teen was developed to assess health literacy in the adolescent population.[12] The REALM-Teen is a word recognition test intended for grades 6 through 12. It allows physicians to recognize adolescent patients that read health-related information below their grade-reading level.[12] This screening tool takes no more than 5 min to administer. Similar to the other screening tools used to assess health literacy in adults, the REALM-Teen has its limitations as it is only available in English.[12]

3.9 Culture, Race, Ethnicity, and Health Literacy

Health literacy is significantly impacting the delivery of healthcare in America. Not only does a patient's age, level of education, language spoken affect the delivery of healthcare, but sociocultural factors, race, and ethnicity also impact the healthcare system.[1,8,23] Culture, race, and ethnicity influence a patient's belief and health practices.[12,23] It is essential that healthcare providers deliver care that is sensitive to the needs of patients from different cultures, race, and ethnicity.[8,23] Achieving cultural competence is a multifaceted project.[8] There has been growing interest in preparing healthcare providers to care for patients with different cultural backgrounds.[8] Despite this interest, only a few studies have been done to examine efforts to educate healthcare providers in cross-cultural care.[8,23] By 2015, it is estimated that over 50% of patients that will be seeking primary care will be of the racial and ethnic minorities.[8] Cultural differences between patients and healthcare providers influence communication, patients' adherence, and health outcome.[23] Certain patients may be viewed as having inadequate health literacy because they have beliefs and practices that are not understood by healthcare professionals. These misunderstandings can lead to negative health outcomes. The role of mistrust in the healthcare system by racial and ethnic minorities is also an important aspect in medical care. African Americans especially carry with them the continuing legacy of the Tuskegee Syphilis Study that contributes to mistrust in the healthcare system.[8, 24,25] A physician's full understanding of this historical experience is necessary in achieving optimal patient–physician encounter.[8] The Society of General Internal Medicine Health Disparities Task Force made recommendations to address the racial and ethnic health. The Task Force recommends examining and understanding patients' attitudes such as mistrust. It was also recommended that the correct skills are needed to effectively communicate across cultures, languages, and literacy levels.

3.10 Health Literacy and Mortality

Patients with inadequate health literacy face enormous obstacles. During the last 15 years researchers have shown that there is some association between inadequate health literacy and poor understanding of chronic diseases, poor self-management skills and underuse of health promoting/disease prevention programs.[5,7]

Unfortunately, patients with inadequate health literacy are at an increased risk for adverse health outcomes including death. One study reported that among community-dwelling adults aged 70–79 years, there was an association between the performance on the REALM and mortality. Worse performance during this screening was associated with higher mortality rates.[5] A prospective cohort study was performed on 3,260 medicare-managed care enrollees in the four previously mentioned US metropolitan areas of Cleveland, Houston, Tampa, and the Ft. Lauderdale/ Miami area.[5] This prospective cohort study was designed to determine if there is a relationship between health literacy and mortality and whether low health literacy independently predicts overall and cause-specific mortality.[5] Health literacy is essential for managing health conditions.[1,12] It is a cornerstone for patient safety in twenty-first-century America. In the study, the participants were of the age 65 years and older. Race/ethnicity, level of education, chronic health conditions, physical and mental health were some of the areas that were assessed. The patients involved in the cohort study were also asked to complete the short form of the TOFHLA, the S-TOFHLA.[5] The S-TOFHLA included two reading passages and four mathematical questions to assess the participants' ability to read and perform numerical tasks. Among the 3,260 participants the number of participants with adequate literacy, marginal literacy, and inadequate literacy were 2,094, 366, and 800 respectively.[5] According to the results of this prospective cohort study, elderly patients with poor health literacy have higher incidence of all cause mortality and cardiovascular death.[5] A participant's health literacy was determined or measured by reading fluency which according to the authors "was a more powerful variable than education for examining the association between SES and health." The study analyzed differences in mortality during a 6-year period. The National Death Index was used to identify the deaths through 2003.[5] Of the 3,260 participants, a total of 815 participants died during an average follow-up period of 67.8 months.[5] For those participants with inadequate health literacy, the crude mortality rate was 39.4% compared with 28.7% in those participants with marginal health literacy. Participants with adequate health literacy had the lowest crude mortality rate of 18.9%.[5] Cardiovascular disease was the cause of death in 11.7% of participants; which accounts for a total of 380 participants. Those participants with inadequate

health literacy had higher rates of mortality secondary to cardiovascular disease (19.3%) as compared to those with marginal health literacy and adequate health literacy whose rates were 16.7 and 7.9% respectively.[5] Although the crude cancer mortality rates were higher in patients with inadequate literacy, multivariate analyses had similar rates. The authors have therefore concluded that "participants with inadequate health literacy had higher risk-adjusted rates of cardiovascular death but not death due to cancer."

The authors explored several possible explanations for the association between health literacy and mortality. Smoking, alcohol use, and physical activity were examined to determine if these behaviors could explain the higher mortality rate among those with inadequate health literacy. Health behaviors were found to be only weakly predictive of mortality.[5] This was also the case when the authors explored the association between the amount of years a participant completed in school and the rate of mortality. In bivariate analyses, years of school completed had a weak association with mortality. In multivariate analyses, the amount of years of school completed did not significantly predict mortality. Since many individuals progress through the school system without meeting desired requirements, the authors also concluded that the number of years completed in school is not a true measure of educational accomplishment.[5] For the elderly, the number of years completed in school does not capture or account for lifelong learning or age-related declines in reading fluency.[12] For this reason, the authors concluded that fluency was a more powerful variable than education.

Inadequate health literacy is associated with poor self-management of chronic diseases such as diabetes and hypertension.[1,6] Medication adherence also becomes affected. To function appropriately in today's healthcare system, patients need to be able to perform numerical tasks. IIIV-positive patients, for example, must be able to follow dosing instructions to properly manage their disease. Use of health promoting/disease prevention measures such as cancer screening and immunization are lower among those with inadequate health literacy.[5] One study done on patients aged 50 years and older concluded that patients with inadequate health literacy were less knowledgeable about colorectal cancer screening.[26] The authors of the July 23 rd issue concluded that the association between health literacy and adverse outcomes such as death is probably secondary to the cumulative effect of multiple causes.[5] Countless numbers of patients are at risk in today's healthcare system because they do not possess adequate health literacy. Inadequate health literacy correlates with decreased knowledge about diseases, decreased medication adherence, increased involvement in risky health behaviors, and a poorer understanding of preventive health measures. Patients with inadequate health literacy are therefore at an increased risk for adverse health outcomes. The adverse health outcome that is most concerning is untimely death, since in most cases, death could be avoided if patients had adequate knowledge about diseases and diagnoses were not delayed. As a result, improvements in communication and possibly improvements in screening will more than likely be necessary to reduce the association between health literacy and mortality.[12,20] According to Baker et al. "To achieve this goal, we must further elucidate the causal pathways linking health literacy and adverse health outcomes and use this information to design more comprehensive and effective interventions."[5]

3.11 Addressing Health Literacy

Inadequate health literacy is surprisingly common in the United States. People of all ages, races, ethnicities, cultures, and education levels are challenged by this problem. During the past decade, the consequence that poor health literacy has had, America's healthcare system has been receiving considerable attention. Many will agree that achieving a health-literate America is a multifaceted project. The AMA became the first national medical organization to adopt a policy that recognizes that there is a causal pathway to how inadequate health literacy negatively affects medical diagnosis and treatment.[12] The AMA's Council on Scientific Affairs, through an Ad-Hoc Committee on Health Literacy, published a report in 1999.[1,12] The report adopted five statements. It was identified in the first statement that limited health literacy is a barrier to medical diagnosis and effective treatment.[12] The remaining statements recommended increasing public awareness, promoting the education of the medical community, supporting assessment of health literacy, and encouraging research on health literacy.[1,12] The joint commission on accreditation of healthcare organizations (JCAHO) added health literacy benchmarks

for hospitals to achieve. JCAHO mandated that hospitals and other health organizations assess patients' knowledge and provide instructions that patients can easily understand.[14] The IOM convened a Committee on Health Literacy. Composed of experts from a wide range of academic disciplines, this committee was created to define the nature and scope of the problem, to identify any obstacles to solving this problem, to assess all the approaches that have been attempted and to identify goals for health literacy and suggest approaches to reach these goals.[4,10] In 2004, the IOM issued a well-written 345-page report, *Health literacy: a prescription to end confusion.* In the words of the IOM report, "efforts to improve quality, reduce cost, and reduce disparities cannot succeed without simultaneous improvements in health literacy."[10] The first finding of the Health Literacy Committee was that health literacy is "based on the interaction of the individuals' skills with health contexts... the healthcare system, the education system and broad social and cultural factors at home, at work and in the community."[10] The healthcare system does not carry sole responsibility for creating a health-literate America. The responsibility must be shared among several sectors in today's society. In the IOM health literacy report recommendations were made to increase both Federal and non-federal funds for research.[10] Future research should focus on improving the health literacy screening methods. Research should also focus on techniques to improve health education.[11] It was also recommended that in order to fulfill accreditation requirements, schools should implement National Health Education standards and funds should be increased to achieve these standards.[10] Professional schools should also incorporate health literacy into their curricula. Private and public healthcare systems should get involved and help to identify ways to improve health literacy in America. Accreditation bodies such as JCAHO should incorporate health literacy assessment in data collection and healthcare information systems.[10]

In the report by the JCAHO titled *"What did the doctor say?": Improving health literacy to protect patient safety* it was identified that inadequate health literacy complicates the communication process between healthcare workers and patients.[27] Effective patient–physician communication has a direct link to improved understanding of diseases, increased medication adherence, and subsequently improved health outcomes. Sociocultural factors complicate the communication process between healthcare providers and patients. During an encounter, three cultures come into play; the culture of the patient, the culture of the physician, and the culture of medicine. America is now in an era where technology is producing numerous breakthrough drug regimens and life-saving treatments.[2] Patients who have a difficult time with health literacy miss out on the life-saving interventions and generally have worse health outcomes. The Joint Commission encourages accredited organizations to ensure patients' understanding by providing information both written and oral in a way that they can understand.[2] Many physicians rely on written health information that are often written at a grade level above most patients' understanding.[1] More than half the written medical information has a readability level at the tenth grade level or higher.[12] In order to facilitate patient understanding, written healthcare materials should be short and simple.[1,12] In a randomized controlled trial the effectiveness of using a low literacy educational handout in increasing pneumococcal vaccine rates was demonstrated.[1] Patients who received this one page instruction sheet written for fifth grade level were four times more likely to discuss the vaccine with their physician.[1,12] It is recommended that materials should be written at the fourth through eighth grade level for the general public to comprehend. The National Institute of Health convened a Plain Language Coordinating Committee that proposed that written materials should be in "plain language." Plain language was defined as "clear writing that tells the reader exactly what the reader needs to know without unnecessary words or expressions."[12] Educational videotapes, pictorial illustrations, and simplified brochures may also improve understanding.[9,12] Oral communication is another strategy that has been proposed. Healthcare providers should avoid using medical jargon and should speak slowly when providing verbal health related information.[1,12] Speaking slowly may prove more beneficial to the elderly since they have a relative decline in cognitive and sensory function. Determining whether or not a patient understands what was said or what was provided in a written form is also very important in a patient–physician encounter. To assess a patient's understanding, physicians should have patients repeat in their own words what was said.[1] This method is called the "teach back" strategy.[1] To facilitate full comprehension, a combination of methods such as oral and written may prove beneficial.

To improve communication some patients may benefit from group sessions. In fact, research has demonstrated that group sessions improve communication and subsequently improve behavioral and health outcomes.[12] Patients with inadequate health literacy often feel embarrassed and by offering this method of communication some patients may find it easier to discuss their health issues. It is essential to deliver care that is sensitive to different races/ethnicities. Culture plays a vital role in shaping an individual's health beliefs and practices. By utilizing educational programs that take into consideration cultural preferences, patients may become more involved and learning will be facilitated.[12] A number of studies have been done to prove the effectiveness of the individualized approach to patient education. At this point in time there is no general consensus that the individualized approach is more effective in improving communication. A one-to-one counseling program was designed for pregnant African American and Hispanic women from WIC (women, infants, and children) who had limited health literacy and smoked.[12] Smoking cessation materials were also provided. Women that were randomized were more likely to quit smoking at the 9-month follow-up session.[12] The relapse rate was also relatively low for ex-smokers.[12]

Parents have a very strong influence on the health of their children because they are responsible for managing health conditions and at the same time preventing adverse health outcomes. Studies that have addressed improving the understanding of adults with low health literacy also have implications that are important for the pediatric population.[12] All parents are required to receive immunization schedules and vaccine information at well-child visits. Since these documents are written at an eleventh grade reading level this poses a threat to those with limited health literacy.[12] In 2005 the American Academy of Pediatrics formed a Health Literacy Project Advisory Committee to address the issue of health literacy as it relates to the pediatric population.[12] As mentioned earlier, approximately 50% of American adults are unable to understand printed healthcare materials.[1] A brief screening test may prove beneficial in identifying the parents that have inadequate health literacy. Adolescent health literacy assessment is also of importance to many researchers. The REALM-Teen allows physicians to assess health literacy in children that are in grades 6 through 12.[12] One disadvantage of the REALM-Teen is that it is only available in English.

It is essential that healthcare workers deliver care that is sensitive to the needs of patients that are from different races/ethnicities and cultures. The authors of a well-written article titled *Viewpoint: cultural competence and the African American experience with healthcare* in the February 2007 issue of Academic Medicine proposed that awareness of historical information of different ethnicities and race may improve communication.[8] The authors identified key influences such as slavery and the Tuskegee syphilis study that have led to African American patients' mistrust in the healthcare system.[8] Patients with inadequate health literacy may have delayed diagnosis of medical conditions because they do not seek medical attention in the early stages of their disease. This could certainly be secondary to some cultural practices that involve the use of home remedies, mistrust in today's healthcare system, or simply because patients have poor understanding about their health.[1,8] Whether patients have inadequate health literacy that is compounded by mistrust in America's healthcare system or not, the authors proposed increasing awareness through cultural education as a method of improving communication in a clinical setting.[8] The Joint Commission also recognizes that addressing culture and even language is essential to quality healthcare.[2] In 2006, the Joint Commission implemented standards that required the documentation of patients' language and communication need by accredited organizations.[2]

At some point in most people's lives, healthcare decisions must be made because they are faced with medical conditions that require medical intervention. Patients with diabetes, for example, need their blood sugars to be properly managed to avoid adverse health outcomes. Widespread improvements in patients' understanding will likely be a necessity if there is to be a reduction in the association between health literacy and adverse health outcomes such as death.[5] Interventions that extend beyond the patient physician encounter should also be addressed.[28] Considering that today's healthcare system has placed a myriad of demands on patients, researchers have proposed multidisciplinary support teams and outreach activities.[28] Recently, management strategies for chronic diseases were developed for those patients with inadequate health literacy.[28] These strategies which included education and follow-up methods for patients with diseases such as diabetes and heart failure appear to be effective.[28]

In a pilot survey study that assessed the knowledge of colorectal cancer screening in patients 50 years and older, it was found that patients with limited health literacy were less likely to be knowledgeable about the screening method.[26] A different approach for improving the education of patients with inadequate health literacy was studied.[12] In a randomized control trial, healthcare providers were trained on screening guidelines for colorectal cancer and on methods to improve communication with patients with limited health literacy.[12] Two thousand VA patients were involved in this trial and were provided with information on colorectal screening via video and a simple and clear pictogram brochure.[12] The trial concluded that patients with inadequate health literacy (health literacy level less than the ninth grade) had an increased likelihood in completing colorectal screening test.[12] Although further studies are recommended on assessing provider training methods, this method may prove beneficial at improving patient understanding and health outcomes.

3.12 Conclusion

The future of America's healthcare system depends on ingenuity and the commitment of necessary resources to improve patient–physician communication and subsequently improve patients' health outcomes. Accepting the fact that health literacy is an issue in the United States is a crucial first step. Healthcare workers need to be more cognizant of the issues associated with inadequate health literacy as they impact patients' morbidity and mortality and America's healthcare costs. Becoming aware of these issues of health literacy as they relate to the patient, to healthcare, and society will enable better planning of care.[27] After accepting that approximately 90 million adults have fair to poor literacy and that 21–23% of adults read at the lowest reading level, the next crucial step is identifying patients with these deficits.[1] No simple method of identifying patients with inadequate health literacy exists and this is complicated by the fact that most are hesitant to disclose their limitations because they are too embarrassed.[1,29] Simply asking a patient for his or her highest level of education attained is not an accurate assessment of the patient's health literacy.[12] One study found a difference of 4.8 grade levels between educational attainment and the actual level the patients read.[12] During the last 15 years, research has focused on several screening methods. Most physicians do not utilize these screening instruments because of time constraints. Others may lack the knowledge on how to address the issue of inadequate health literacy when they indentify a patient with this deficit.[12] During the past decade, the magnitude of inadequate health literacy and consequences it has had on America's healthcare system have been receiving attention. Although research is now gaining momentum the pace is not fast enough and the scope is not broad enough.[10] The time is now to reach a resolution. We are certainly in an era where there are drug regimens and technology that can save patients' lives. There should be no reason, therefore, that countless numbers of patients have poor health outcomes and are dying from health conditions that can be cured or at least treated. One study concluded that the crude mortality rate of patients with inadequate health literacy was highest at almost 40% relative to those participants with marginal and adequate health literacy which were 28.7 and 18.9% respectively.[5] Patients with inadequate health literacy have a vast array of communication difficulties and therefore are less likely to effectively self-manage diseases or utilize preventive services.[1,6,14] Physicians need to be aware of certain behaviors that are suggestive of inadequate literacy skills such as frequently missing appointments, noncompliance with medication, incompletely filling out forms, misspellings, need for assistance, and mimicking others.[1,12] Physicians also need to evaluate themselves on their own literacy and identify areas that need improvement. One area that must be improved is the understanding of different cultures and ethnicities. Effective communication across different cultures and ethnicities is directly linked to improved patient satisfaction and increased adherence.[23] Adverse health outcomes that may be associated with inappropriate treatment of chronic diseases such as diabetes and hypertension can be avoided if there is effective communication between patients and physicians. Both direct and indirect causal pathways that link inadequate health literacy to adverse health outcomes must be further explored and this information should be used to design interventions.[5]

Pediatric health is dependent on the health literacy of parents/caregivers. By addressing the communication between parents/caregivers and physicians, adverse health outcomes that affect children may be avoided. The American Academy of pediatrics in 2005 formed a committee to address issues of inadequate health literacy and how it relates to the pediatric population.[12] In the well-written article *Health literacy and pediatric health* by Yin, MD et al. the American academy of pediatrics health literacy project advisory committee was introduced.[12] The article stated that this committee is in the process of developing an agenda to address the challenges that parents with inadequate health literacy may face and how this affects the health of America's children.[12] Among the projects proposed by the committee were parent handouts in English and Spanish and health literacy guidebook for pediatricians. Although the committee is developing an agenda to address the impact of low literacy and the pediatric population there is limited research on this topic.[12]

The 2004 IOM report suggested that the healthcare system should not be solely responsible for addressing health literacy in America but instead other areas of society such as the education system should play a vital role. Direct involvement of patients should also be encouraged. In developing educational materials, a patient's direct involvement may empower him or her to, for example, avoid risky behaviors, use preventive services, and subsequently improve his or her own health.[30] Future research should explore the usefulness of screening and address the improvements in educational techniques. Certainly, the increased cost associated with inadequate health literacy needs effective intervention.[11] Now is the time to make this happen. The issues associated with this health literacy epidemic should not be ignored. Awareness must be increased to effectively achieve a health-literate America.

References

1. Keenan J, Safeer R. Health literacy: the gap between physicians and patients. *Am Fam Phys*. 2005;72:463–468
2. Murphy–Knoll L. Low health literacy puts patients at risk. *J Nurs Care Qual*. 2007;22:205–209
3. Anon. Health literacy. Report of council on scientific affairs. *JAMA*. 1999;281:552
4. Kindig DA, Nielsen-Bohlman L, Panzer AM. Health literacy: a prescription to end confusion. *N Engl J Med*. 2005; 352:947–948
5. Baker DW, Gazmararian JA, et al Health literacy and mortality among elderly persons. *Arch Intern Med*. 2007; 167: 1503–1509
6. Baker DW, Gazmararian JA, Wolf MS. Health literacy and functional health status among older adults. *Arch Intern Med*. 2005;165:1946–1952

7. Wallace L. Patients' health literacy skills: the missing demographic variable in primary care research. *Ann Fam Med.* 2006;4:85–86

8. Eiser AR, Ellis G. Viewpoint: cultural competence and the African American experience with health care: the case for specific content in cross–cultural education. *Acad Med.* 2007;82(2):176–183

9. Marcus EN. The silent epidemic – the health effects of illiteracy. *N Engl J Med.* 2006;355:339–341

10. Kindig DA, Parker RM. Beyond the institute of medicine health literacy report: are the recommendations being taken seriously. *J Gen Intern Med.* 2006;21(8):891–892

11. Kellerman R, Rudd R, et al Health literacy: report of the council on scientific affairs. Ad Hoc Committee on Health Literacy for the Council on Scientific Affairs, American Medical Association. *JAMA.* 1999;282:525–527

12. Dreyer BP, Forbis SG, Yin HS. Health literacy and pediatric health. *Curr Probl Pediatr Adolesc Health Care.* 2007;37: 258–286

13. Bindman AB, Castro C, Schillinger D, et al Physician communication with diabetic patients who have low health literacy. *Arch Intern Med.* 2003;163:83–90

14. Baker DW, Nurss JR, et al Relationship of functional health literacy to patients' knowledge of their chronic disease. A study of patients with hypertension and diabetes. *Arch Intern Med.* 1998;158:166–172

15. Betancourt JR, Bowles J, et al Recommendations for teaching about racial and ethnic disparities in health and health care. *Ann intern Med.* 2007;147(9):654–665

16. Baer J, Kutner REF, Greenberg E. National assessment of Adult Literacy (NAAL). A first look at the literacy of America's adults in 21st century. Available at: <http://nces.cd.gov/naal>; 2009 Accessed 16.04.09

17. Baker DW, Gazmararian JA, Fehrenbach SN, et al Health literacy among medicare enrollees in a managed care organization. *JAMA.* 1999;281:545–551

18. Satterfield S, Sudore RL, Yaffe K, et al Limited Literacy and mortality in the elderly: the health, aging and body composition study. *J Gen Intern Med.* 2006;21:806

19. Bass PF, Davis TC, Wolf MS, et al Literacy and misunderstanding prescription drug labels. *Ann Intern Med.* 2006; 145:887

20. Weiss BD, Mays MZ, Martz W, et al Quick assessment of literacy in primary care: the newest vital sign. *Ann Fam Med.* 2005;3:514–522

21. Grumbach K, Piette J, Schillinger D, et al Association of health literacy with diabetes outcomes. *JAMA.* 2002; 288:475

22. Baker D, Blazer DG, Gazmararian J, et al A multivariate analysis of factors associated with depression. Evaluating the role of health literacy as a potential contributor. *Arch Intern Med.* 2000;160:3307–3314

23. Flores G. Culture and the patient–physician relationship: achieving cultural competency in health care. *J Pediatr.* 2000;136:14

24. Thomas SB, Quinn SC. Public health then and now. The Tuskegee Syphilis Study, 1932 to 1972: implications for HIV education and AIDS risk education programs in black community. *Am J Public Health.* 1991;81:1498–1504

25. White RM. Misinformation and misbeliefs in the Tuskegee Study of Untreated Syphilis fuel mistrust in the health care system. *J Natl Med Assoc.* 2005;97:1566–1573

26. Brownlee CD, McCoy TP, Miller DP, et al The effect of health literacy on knowledge and receipt of colorectal cancer screening: a survey study. *BMC Fam Pract.* 2007;8:16

27. Ross J. Health literacy and its influence on patient safety. *J Peri Anes Nurs.* 2007;22:220 222

28. Bennett L, Davis TC, Wolf MS, et al Literacy, self efficacy, and HIV medication adherence. *Patient Educ Couns.* 2007; 65:253 260

29. Parikh NS, Parker RM, Nurss JR, et al Shame and health literacy: the unspoken connection. *Patient Educ Couns.* 1996;27:33 39

30. Comings JP, Rudd RE. Learner developed materials: an empowering product. *Health Educ Q.* 1994;21:313–327

Domestic Violence, Abuse, and Neglect: Indicators for Dermatology

4

Jina P. Lewallen and Susan R. Adams

4.1 Introduction

This chapter will discuss the prevalence of domestic violence and abuse and/or neglect of patients and the dermatologic indicators for assessment, diagnosis, and treatment. This chapter includes the following:

- A definition and view of domestic violence, abuse, and/or neglect
- Review of current literature to include national and global statistics that demonstrate the prevalence of these issues
- Mandated reporting laws and process
- Assessment and diagnosis for the dermatologist
- Multidisciplinary approach in treatment
- Case studies
- Follow-up issues

4.2 Definitions

We need to begin with a definition of domestic violence, abuse (physical and sexual), and neglect. To understand sexual abuse and domestic violence, we must first agree on what these are. The United States Centers for Disease Control and Prevention[1] defines domestic violence as:

> Actual or threatened physical or sexual violence, or psychological/emotional abuse by a spouse, ex-spouse, boyfriend/girlfriend, ex-boyfriend/ex-girlfriend, or date. Some of the common terms that are used to describe intimate partner

violence are domestic abuse, spouse abuse, domestic violence, courtship violence, battering, marital rape and date rape.

Domestic violence is a pattern of abusive and threatening behaviors that may include physical, emotional, economic, and sexual violence as well as intimidation, isolation, and coercion. The purpose of domestic violence is to establish and exert power and control over another; men most often use it against their intimate partners, such as current or former spouses, girlfriends, or dating partners. While other forms of violence within the family are also serious, this chapter will address the unique characteristics of violence against women in their intimate relationships.

Domestic violence is a behavior that is learned through observation and reinforcement in both the family and society. It is not caused by genetics or illness. Domestic violence is repeated because it works. Domestic violence allows the perpetrator to gain control of the victim through fear and intimidation. Gaining the victim's compliance, even temporarily, reinforces the perpetrator's use of these tactics of control. More importantly, however, the perpetrator's abusive behavior is reinforced by the socially sanctioned belief that men have the right to control women in relationships and the right to use force to ensure that control.[2]

Sexual abuse refers to any sexual activity perpetrated against another person, against their will or without consent. Child sexual abuse is defined as sexual violation of a child who cannot give consent.

In the United States and several countries, medical and social service professionals, along with law enforcement and the clergy, are mandated by law to report any suspected abuse or neglect to law officers. After the report is made, a follow-up to determine abuse or neglect is made, usually within 24–72 h. Failure to report by professionals can result in loss of

J.P. Lewallen (✉)
Department of Geriatrics,
University of Arkansas for Medical Sciences,
Little Rock, AR, USA
e-mail: lewallenjinap@uams.edu

R.A. Norman (ed.), *Common Treatments in Preventive Dermatology*,
DOI 10.1007/978-0-85729-853-9_4, © Springer-Verlag London Limited 2012

licensure or privilege to work in that profession. Dermatologists fall within this category.

Practitioners should also be aware of the importance of informed consent when treating patients. It is crucial in the development of trust in creating the therapeutic alliance. Informed consent in relation to abuse cases includes an understanding between patient and practitioner regarding the role of mandated reporting. This should be in addition to standard disclosure and understanding statements related to treatment options and risks.

Other types of violence perpetrated against women and children can be seen in child and elder abuse. There are a smaller percentage of men who are victims of domestic abuse and the number of male children is significant in cases of sexual abuse.

4.3 Common Characteristics of Victims

Victims may share common characteristics regardless of age or sex. They are often overwhelmed by feelings of helplessness and dependency. Presentation of anxiety or anger, along with multiple physical complaints, may be present during the diagnostic interview. Victims may feel responsible for the abuse or neglect and will often provided detailed explanations for the perpetrators actions. Typically, symptoms of depression and low self-esteem will also be a factor. In addition to the injuries sustained, emotional trauma and damage persists long after physical health is restored. It is common for children and adults to "try harder" to prevent future attacks. Understanding the futility of this mission is difficult for victims to comprehend.

4.3.1 Children

Federal legislation provides a foundation for the states by identifying a minimum set of acts or behaviors that define child abuse and neglect. The federal child abuse prevention and treatment act (CAPTA),[3] as amended by the Keeping Children and Families Safe Act of 2003 defines child abuse and neglect as, at minimum:

> Any recent act or failure to act on the part of a parent or caretaker which results in death, serious physical or emotional harm, sexual abuse or exploitation; or An act or failure to act which presents an imminent risk of serious harm.

This definition of child abuse and neglect refers specifically to parents and other caregivers. A "child" under this definition generally means a person who is under the age of 18 or who is not an emancipated minor. Children with special needs are at a higher risk of abuse or neglect. Many times children will wear the history of their trauma including scars, physical abnormalities, or disabilities. Head injury is a major cause of death and permanent disability for children under the age of two; therefore, special attention should be given to internal ear and eye exams. Bones and joints are manipulated to assess for tenderness and range of motion. Addressing eating patterns, sleeping patterns, problems swallowing, and mastery of age-appropriate tasks are also areas for assessment.

4.3.2 Elder Abuse and Domestic Violence

Elder domestic abuse is a pattern of violence started earlier in life that has persisted in later years. It may also begin in later life due to strains of retirement, disability, or illness that comes in aging years. Like domestic violence in early years, the perpetrators are usually male.

Elder sexual abuse is any nonconsensual contact with an older person. This includes fondling, oral, anal, vaginal sex, pornography, and other sexual acts meant to demean, injure, or mental or emotionally trauma as a result of contact.

Physical abuse is any physical contact that results in injury, pain, or impairment. This includes hitting, kicking, biting, and inappropriate restraint of an elderly person.

Psychological abuse and financial abuse are also of importance and should be noted. According to the national incident study on elder abuse:

- Female elders are abused at a higher rate than males, after accounting for their larger proportion in the aging population.
- Our oldest elders (80 years and over) are abused and neglected at 2–3 times their proportion of the elderly population.
- In almost 90% of the elder abuse and neglect incidents with a known perpetrator, the perpetrator is a family member, and two-thirds of the perpetrators are adult children or spouses.

4.3.3 *Warning Signs*

It is important for every healthcare provider to be aware of and act on signs and symptoms of abuse while creating a safe environment for the elderly person to report without fear of continued mistreatment from family and/or caregivers.

The National Elder Abuse Incidence Study[4] prepared for the administration for children and families and the administration on aging in the US Department of Health and Human Services gives the signs and symptoms shown in Table 4.1 to assist healthcare professionals in what to look for when investigating possible abuse of children and elderly persons.

4.4 Mandatory Reporting

Victims of domestic abuse or sexual abuse need immediate medical care. In the United States, healthcare providers are mandated by state laws to report suspected abuse or neglect of any patient they treat.

According to the child welfare information gateway,[5] all states, the District of Columbia, the Commonwealth of Puerto Rico, and the US territories of American Samoa, Guam, the Northern Mariana Islands, and the Virgin Islands have statutes identifying mandatory reporters of child maltreatment. A mandatory reporter is a person who is required by law to make a report of child maltreatment under specific circumstances. Approximately 48 states, the District of Columbia, Puerto Rico, and the territories have designated individuals, typically by professional group, who are mandated by law to report child maltreatment. Individuals typically designated as mandatory reporters have frequent contact with children. Such individuals may include:

- Physicians
- Social workers
- School personnel
- Healthcare workers
- Mental health professionals
- Childcare providers
- Medical examiners or coroners
- Law enforcement officers

The same applies for all ages of suspected abuse or neglect victims. Each state determines who is a mandated reporter. Failure to report, in many states, can result in fines, penalties, and loss of licensure to practice. Check with your local authority.

Reporting is mandatory whenever a healthcare professional suspects domestic violence, abuse, or neglect, whether or not it is proven. Some professionals are very sensitive about reporting suspected abuse for fear of misreporting or repercussions over unproved reports. However, the law protects mandatory reporters from prosecution if the report is not proven. It is important to remember that you must report and failure to do so can affect your practice in the future.

4.5 Common Characteristics of Abusers

Along with an awareness of possible victims, practitioners should also be cognizant of possible perpetrators as well. It is not unusual for the abuser to bring the victim to medical appointments and to insist on being part of the interview.

Persons who abuse lack control over aggressive impulses that lead to explosive behavior. The offenders will often explain their behavior as a form of "discipline" and necessary. Emotional immaturity is a common problem, as is the inability to process situations in an appropriate manner. Narcissism is also a common characteristic that leads to difficulty in engaging and maintaining adult relationships. This egocentric view interferes with the abusers' ability to recognize the needs of others. They may also view their potential victims as objects responsible for meeting their needs.

Persons who abuse have a tendency to be suspicious of everyone with whom they are in contact. On some level, there is recognition that their behavior is abnormal in relation to society's expectations and they fear exposure. There are no obvious signs of mental illness, substance abuse, or related symptoms that can easily establish the identity of an offender, so it is important to be aware of indicators in order to obtain additional information about your patients and their situations.

4.6 Role of Healthcare Provider

The role of the healthcare provider in detecting and preventing abuse begins with the first look or assessment of the patient. For dermatology, assessment of

Table 4.1 Warning signs of abuse and neglect in children and the elderly

General
Frequent unexplained crying
Unexplained fear of or suspicion of particular person(s) in the home
Bruises, black eyes, welts, lacerations, and rope marks
Bone fractures, broken bones, and skull fractures
Open wounds, cuts, punctures, untreated injuries, and injuries in various stages of healing
Stains, dislocations, and internal injuries/bleeding
Broken eyeglasses/frames
Physical signs of being subjected to punishment and signs of being restrained
Laboratory findings of medication overdose or underutilization of prescribed drugs
An elder's report of being hit, slapped, kicked, or mistreated
An elder's sudden change in behavior
A caregiver's refusal to allow visitors to see an elder alone
Sexual abuse
Bruises around the breasts or genital area
Unexplained venereal disease or genital infections
Unexplained vaginal or anal bleeding
Torn, stained, or bloody underclothing
An elder's report of being sexually assaulted or raped
Emotional and psychological abuse
Emotional upset or agitation
Extreme withdrawal and noncommunication or nonresponsiveness
An elder's report of being verbally or emotionally mistreated
Neglect
Dehydration, malnutrition, untreated bedsores, and poor personal hygiene
Unattended or untreated health problems
Hazardous or unsafe living conditions (e.g., improper wiring, no heat or no running water)
Unsanitary or unclean living conditions (e.g., dirt, fleas, lice on person, soiled bedding, fecal/urine smell, inadequate clothing)
An elder's report of being neglected
Abandonment
The desertion of an elder at a hospital, nursing facility, or other similar institution
The desertion of an elder at a shopping center or other public location
An elder's own report of being abandoned
Self-neglect
Dehydration, malnutrition, untreated or improperly attended medical conditions, and poor personal hygiene
Hazardous or unsafe living conditions (e.g., improper wiring, no indoor plumbing, no heat, or no running water)
Unsanitary or unclean living quarters (e.g., animal/insect infestation, no functioning toilet, fecal/urine smell)
Inappropriate and/or inadequate clothing, lack of necessary medical aids (e.g., eyeglasses, hearing aid, dentures)
Grossly inadequate housing or homelessness

bruises, cuts, and abrasions can be relevant in the diagnosis of a skin disease or condition, or of suspected abuse. There are many skin conditions that mimic signs of abuse and will be discussed later in the chapter.

One of the most difficult problems caused by these family dynamics is treatment noncompliance. As noted, offenders may be very suspicious of any medical professional attempting to engage the victim. They may discourage the patient from keeping return appointments or refuse to allow private interviews with the victim. They may have multiple caregivers in order to avoid arousing suspicion.

4.6.1 Patient Interviews

When working with patients, interviews should be non-threatening and nonjudgmental. It is easy to become part of the abusive system rather than a possible haven. Beginning the interview by asking general, nonthreatening questions will help the client feel more at ease. Making basic inquires into patients needs will indicate the willingness to listen and open the doorway to more detailed communication. Some victims will have a desire to discuss the situation quickly while others may choose to be more cautious in their revelations. Once rapport has been established, it will be necessary to address the injuries and their possible origins. Patients will need to know they will have some form of protection if abuse is revealed to the physician. Accurate referral information should be maintained in the office.

When evaluating patients for possible abuse, there are several factors that should be noted in developing an assessment[6] including

- Nonverbal communication between patient and caregiver, partner, or parent
- Verbal communication between patient and caregiver, partner, or parent
- Body language of all persons involved
- Balance of communication between patient and practitioner and caregiver, partner, or parent
- Dominant or submissive behavior of patient and caregiver, partner, or parent
- Effectual responses to interview material
- Ability to answer questions directly vs. subject changes and evasive, tangential, or irrelevant answers
- Comfort levels of individuals during interview

Practitioners must fully understand the implications of abuse and mandated reporting and be competent to safeguard the patient if abuse is suspected.

4.7 Statistics on Abuse, Neglect, and Violence

Although men can be victims of domestic violence, abuse, or neglect, reports indicate that while males have a higher incident of abuse as children, as adults they are rarely a reported victim. Many potential male victims do not report for various reasons. Some men feel they could have prevented the abuse; others victimized by another male, fear to reveal intimate details of their sexual orientation. In the elderly, men may fail to report because they are not cognitively aware that they have been mistreated. In this case, professionals should take extra care in assessing for potential abuse. The same holds true for any elderly or mentally disabled person.

Up to 44% of American women have experienced some type of domestic violence during their lives, either as a witness or as a victim.[7, 8]

The prevalence of violence, abuse, and neglect for women and children is not limited to the United States. Globally, that number is even higher; one out of three women reported being beaten, raped, or abused emotionally or economically during her lifetime.[9] Many of the women reported witnessing or being a victim of abuse as children.

Outcomes for women and children victims are many[10]:

- More than three women are murdered every day by husbands or boyfriends as a result of domestic violence.
- One in five high school females report being abused sexually or physically by a dating partner.
- Half of the men who abuse their wives also abuse their children.
- Three in four 18-year-old women reported rape or physical assault by a dating partner, cohabitating partner, or spouse; corroborating police reports that showed reported attacks by an acquaintance were higher than assault by a stranger.

Globally, domestic violence is dependent on definition of cultural norms and laws. Many countries do not have laws or enforce laws that deal with domestic violence as they find it culturally acceptable. Some of these practices are seen in the statistics for global violence.

Global statistics vary, but indicate prevalence for abuse through sex and human trafficking, increased rates of HIV and AIDS in women and children, murder, genital mutilation, and an increase in hospitalizations for women and children as the result of domestic, physical, or sexual violence.[11]

In healthcare practice, cultural norms must be considered in assessment and treatment of suspected abuse. While many countries agree on the definition of domestic violence, sexual abuse, and neglect, some practice violence as part of their culture.

An example of this can be seen in the practice of female genital mutilation (FGM), a cultural practice many would consider physical or sexual abuse of female children.[12]

Each year at least two million girls face the risk of genital mutilation, most of who are between 2 and 8 years old. About 85–114 million females worldwide have mutilated genitalia. Most of these females reside in Africa. They encounter pain, trauma, and often, physical complications (e.g., bleeding, infections, and death). FGM consists of clitoridectomy (partial or total removal of the clitoris and/or the labia minora) or infibulation (total removal of the clitoris, partial or total removal of the labia minora, and incisions in the labia majora).

FGM is a cultural, not religious, tradition which is used to prepare girls for womanhood. Muslims, Christians, some animists, and one Jewish sect practice FGM, but none of these religions require FGM. It is used to perpetuate women's second-class status. FGM enhances the sexual pleasure of men while genitally mutilated women sense little or no sexual pleasure. This denial of sexual pleasure can have psychological effects on women. These women therefore become sexual objects and reproductive vehicles for men.

The FGM practitioners vary by area and include traditional birth attendants, female laypeople, physicians and other trained health personnel, and women leaders. African women created the Inter-African Committee Against Traditional Practices Affecting the Health of Women and Children in 1984, which serves as the basis for global action against FGM. African immigrants in developed countries have taken the practice of FGM with them. Women in these countries have brought FGM to the fore and are pressing for laws against it.

Protection from physical and sexual abuse, such as FGM, is a child's right. Information on prevalence, physical, and psychological effects, and religious requirements are needed to take action against FGM.

Legal remedies include international action and national law. Each country's mass communication systems and popular culture should be engaged in spreading information about FGM and in generating discussions on FGM.

In the United States, FMG is considered child abuse and is reportable to legal and social services agencies.

A report[13] that surveyed and analyzed doctors' reporting records found that one-third of the surveyed doctors did not keep a record on domestic violence reported by patients, nor did they report much support, advice, or resources to those who did report being a victim. Only 10% of doctors in the survey reported giving any information on where patients could seek assistance. A third reported that they were not confident about counseling patients who reported domestic abuse. This report demonstrates the need for physicians and other healthcare professionals to get training and be aware of mandated reporting laws.

Many healthcare settings have diverse populations. Patients come from different racial, ethnic, or cultural backgrounds and practitioners need to be aware of cultural norms or differences.

In many cultures, traditional treatments are used before seeking professional medical treatments. Healthcare practitioners should be knowledgeable about certain cultural practices as they can also resemble indicators of abuse. When assessing patients for diagnoses, the practitioner may observe what looks like abuse indicators, so a complete history of the patient, including cultural norms, is indicated.

Some examples that apply to dermatology can be seen in therapeutic burning (moxibustion), cupping, coin rubbing, and pinching.

Moxibustion, or therapeutic burning, is a folk remedy used in Southwest Asia and parts of Africa. Dot and patterned burns on the abdominal area, arms, and legs are thought to correlate to the internal energy channels on the skin. In Korean culture, moxibustion is used to correct the disharmony in the body due to illness. The yin and the yang are rebalanced and the patient is considered healed.

Cupping is a very common folk treatment. A piece of cotton or material is set afire in the bottom of a glass or cup and the open mouth of the vessel is quickly placed on the patient's back. The heat and suction produces a bruise or welt and sometimes a burn. The procedure may be repeated up and down the back of the patient. The cupped areas are believed to draw out fever and illness. Many people who go for cupping treatments believe it will eliminate toxins through breathing and through the skin. It is believed that cupping draws out any illness in the body, leaving the patient healthier overall.

Coin rubbing or coining is another common folk remedy for releasing illness or fever from the body. In the traditional technique, a coin is dipped in oil or mentholated cream and rubbed across the skin to produce welts or burns. This practice is believed to restore balance in the sick patient by withdrawing illness.

In addition to cupping and coining, many Asian cultures and medicinal practices include pinching. The treatment involves pinching the neck, bridge of the nose, and other areas of the skin where the illness is believed to originate. The pinching is severe enough to cause dermabrasion or bruising to the skin. This practice is believed to draw out the bad force or illness and restores body balance.

Other mimickers of abuse include dermatological conditions unrelated to previous folk treatments. Dermatitis as a result of irritants, seborrheic dermatitis, pinworms, and scabies can be misdiagnosed by general practitioners. Referral to dermatology specialists is warranted.

Other skin conditions that may mimic abuse warrant a closer evaluation by the practitioner. There are many incidents where skin conditions may mimic abuse[14]:

- Genital warts
- Pigmented vulvar hamartomas
- Darier's disease
- Lichen sclerosus
- Crohn's disease
- Localized varicella or zoster infection
- Pseudoverrucous papules
- Hemangiomas
- Urethral prolapse
- Allergic contact dermatitis

4.8 Assessment and Diagnoses for Dermatology

In assessing the patient for suspected abuse or neglect, the dermatologist needs to conduct a thorough examination of the patient, keep accurate documentation, obtain photographs, and ensure the patient's safety during the process.

For bruising, True petechiae and purpura, infections, group A streptococcal infections, Lichen sclerosus, vascular malformities, phytophotodermatitis.

Mongolian spots, urticaria/angioedema, pernio to folk medicine remedies such as "cupping" and Cao gio or coin rubbing, both used to "draw out fever and disease."

For mimicking burns: impetigo, diaper dermatitis, pernio, chemical burns from over-the-counter treatments such as analgesic balm, sunburn can be observed as inflicted burns and reported as abuse.

In cases as a result of abuse, team care is absolute in diagnosing, treating, reporting, and follow up for the victim. Team care needs to include healthcare providers, social services, legal authorities to ensure the safety of the patient, especially in abuse cases involving minors or elderly who are most often vulnerable.

4.9 Prevalence

A broad view and understanding of the prevalence of domestic violence, abuse, and neglect can be found in Bureau of Justice statistics[15] (Table 4.2). On average since 2001, for nonfatal intimate partner violence, about one-third of female and male victims reported that they were physically attacked (Table 4.3) while two-thirds said that they were threatened with attack, including threats with a weapon and threats to kill (Table 4.4). Half of the females suffered an injury from their victimization. Forty-four percent suffered minor injuries while 5% were seriously injured; 3% were raped or sexually assaulted (Table 4.5). More than one-third of the male victims were injured: 36% with minor injuries and 4% with major injuries (Table 4.6). Less than one-fifth of victims reporting an injury sought treatment following the injury (Table 4.7).

Table 4.2 Average annual percent of threats, attempted attacks, and physical attacks in nonfatal intimate partner victimization, 2001–2005

Type of violence	Percent of victims of intimate partner violence	
	Male	Female
Attempt or threat	67.2	66.3
Physically attacked	32.8	33.7
	100	100

Table 4.3 Average annual percent of attacks, by type, in nonfatal intimate partner violent crime, 2001–2005

Type of attack	Percent of victims of nonfatal intimate partner violence who were attacked	
	Male	Female
Raped	7.2	0.8[a]
Sexual assault	1.9	0.9
Attacked with firearm	0.5[a]	–
Attacked with knife	2.5	8[a]
Hit by thrown object	2.1	4.5[a]
Attacked with other weapon	0.8[a]	1.8[a]
Hit, slapped, knocked down	62.7	62.2
Grabbed, held, tripped	54.9	26

"–" Information is not provided because the small number of cases is insufficient for reliable estimates
[a]Based on ten or fewer sample cases

Table 4.4 Average annual percent of threats, by type and gender, in nonfatal intimate partner violence crime, 2001–2005

Type of threat	Percent of victims of nonfatal intimate partner violence, 2001–2005	
	Male	Female
Threatened to kill	26.9	15.1[a]
Threatened to rape	0.5[a]	–
Threatened with harm	59.3	55.3
Threatened with a weapon	17.6	22.9
Threw object at victim	7.5	7.4[a]
Followed/surrounded victim	5.9	1.8[a]
Tried to hit, slap, or knock down victim	14.1	12.6[a]

Note: detail may not add to total because victims may have reported more than one type of threat
"–" Information is not provided because the small number of cases is insufficient for reliable estimates
[a]Based on ten or fewer sample cases

Table 4.5 Average annual number and percent of injuries sustained by female victims as a result of nonfatal intimate partner violence, 2001–2005

Intimate partner victim	Average annual	
	Number	Percent
Total	510,970	100
Not injured	248,805	48.7
Injured	262,170	51.3
Serious injury	25,710	5
Gunshot wound	595	0.1[a]
Knife wounds	4,940	1[a]
Internal injuries	3,440	0.7[a]
Broken bones	12,155	2.4
Knocked unconscious	3,730	0.7[a]
Other serious injuries	855	0.2[a]
Rape/sexual assault without additional injuries	13,350	2.6
Minor injuries only	222,670	43.6
Injuries unknown	435	0.1[a]

Note: total may not add to 100% due to rounding
[a]Based on ten or fewer sample cases

Table 4.6 Average annual number and percent of injuries sustained by male victims as a result of nonfatal intimate partner violence, 2001–2005

	Average annual	
	Number	Percent
Total intimate partner victims	104,820	100
Not injured	61,285	58.5
Injured	43,540	41.5
Serious injury	4,335	4.1[a]
Minor injuries only	38,050	36.3
Rape/sexual assault without other injuries	580	0.6[a]
Injuries unknown	570	0.5[a]

Note: detail may not add to totals due to rounding
[a]Based on ten or fewer sample cases

4.9.1 Costs of Violence-Related Injury in America

The costs of assessing, diagnosing, and treating domestic abuse are high. According to the Centers for Disease Control and Prevention[16]:

- Americans suffer 16,800 homicides and 2.2 million medically treated injuries due to interpersonal violence annually, at a cost of $37 billion ($33 billion in productivity losses, $4 billion in medical treatment).
- The cost of self-inflicted injuries (suicide and attempted suicide) is $33 billion annually ($32 billion in productivity losses, $1 billion in medical costs).

Table 4.7 Average annual percent of medical treatment sought as a result of nonfatal intimate partner violence, by gender, 2001–2005

	Average annual (%)	
	Male	Female
Not injured	48.7	58.5
Injured	51.3	41.5
Injured, not treated	32.8	27.9
Treated for injury	18.5	13.1
At scene or home	8.3	9.8
Doctor's office or clinic	1.3	0.6 [a]
Hospital	8.7	2.8[a]
Not admitted	8.4	2.8[a]
Admitted	0.3	–
Other locale	0.2	–
Don't know	–	0.5[a]

"–" Information is not provided because the small number of cases was insufficient for reliable estimates Note: detail may not add to totals due to rounding
[a]Based on ten or fewer sample cases

- People aged 15–44 years comprise 44% of the population, but account for nearly 75% of injuries and 83% of costs due to interpersonal violence.

4.9.2 Result of Violence-Related Injury[17]

- The average cost per homicide was $1.3 million in lost productivity and $4,906 in medical costs.
- The average cost per case for a nonfatal assault resulting in hospitalization was $57,209 in lost productivity and $24,353 in medical costs.
- The average cost per case of suicide is $1 million lost productivity and $2,596 in medical costs.
- The average cost for a nonfatal self-inflicted injury was $9,726 in lost productivity and $7,234 in medical costs.
- Economic costs provide, at best, an incomplete measure of the toll of violence. Victims of violence are more likely to experience a broad range of mental and physical health problems not reflected in these estimates from posttraumatic stress disorder to depression, cardiovascular disease, and diabetes.

4.10 Identification and Assessment of the Patient

In healthcare settings, many victims of domestic, physical, or sexual abuse present themselves for other medical issues or with unexplained or poorly explained injuries.

Some patients present with chronic pain complaints, some with bruising, scratches, or burns that are not consistent with accidental injury. Patients who are victims of abuse may cover their common sites of injury such as arms, neck, breasts, chest, and abdomen with clothing, many times inappropriate for the weather. An example of this can be seen in patients coming in with turtleneck or long-sleeved shirts in summer. Hats, gloves, and scarves are also commonly used.

In assessing for physical injuries in the healthcare setting it is important to make the patient feel safe. Patients are often reluctant to report abuse or violence for fear of retribution from abuser, separation from abuser, and uncertainty of belief from the provider assessing them and to uncertainty of what will happen to them if they report. This is prevalent in domestic violence as the perpetrator of the abuse is a spouse who has isolated their partner from family and friends and made her dependent on him for economic and emotional support.

4.10.1 Universal Guidelines

These guidelines are globally recognized as a complete assessment for diagnosis and charting procedures for evidence for mandated reporting.[18]

4.10.1.1 Physical Examination

All healthcare providers should implement routine physical exam techniques that ensure accurate medical diagnosis:

- Central distribution of injury: face, neck, throat, chest, abdomen, genitals
- Bilateral distribution of injury to multiple areas
- Contusions, lacerations, abrasions, human bites, or no evidence of physical trauma despite subjective complaint by patient/victim
- Delay between onset of injury and presentation for treatment

- Multiple injuries in various stages of healing
- Extent or type of injury inconsistent with patient's explanation
- Evidence of alcohol or drug abuse
- Evidence of rape
- Repeated chronic injuries
- Chronic pain, psychogenic pain, or pain due to diffuse trauma without visible evidence
- Documentation of pertinent negative findings should address all subjective complaints for which there is no physical evidence
- With the patient's permission, photographs should be obtained of visible injuries

Any assessment for domestic violence should be included as part of psychosocial and mental health assessments. The stress of domestic violence may aggravate psychiatric disorders. Mental health disorders can be exacerbated by domestic violence, sexual abuse, or neglect. Some mental health reactions can be observed and assessed in the patient as:

- Suicidal thoughts and attempts
- Depression
- Feelings of helplessness
- Substance abuse
- Posttraumatic stress disorder
- Psychoses

In addition, healthcare providers should be especially alert to injuries and indicators during pregnancy including:

- Injuries, particularly to the breasts, abdomen, and genital area.
- Substance abuse, poor nutrition, depression, and late or sporadic access to prenatal care.
- "Spontaneous" abortions, miscarriages, and premature labor.
- Rapid heartbeat, asthma, and reported inability to sleep.

4.10.1.2 Charting

Healthcare providers should make a complete, legible record/chart of their findings. *The reporting form is no substitute for complete documentation in the medical record.* This chart should include:

- A detailed description of patient injuries: type, extent, age, location, and the use of a body chart when applicable (see resources at the end of the chapter).
- Photographs of patient injuries. The patient should be informed that the photographs are to be used as possible evidence and give permission.
- The maintenance of physical evidence. Forensic nurses and technicians collect physical evidence, and social services are available for emotional assessment and support during the process of examination.
- The inclusion of relevant past medical history: history of falls, "accident prone" injuries; social history: overly concerned partner; history of substance abuse (including alcohol) by patient or partner; and sexual history: history of sexually transmitted diseases or rape.
- All charts should include comments by the healthcare providers as to whether the explanation offered for the injury adequately explains the injury.
- The patient's own words, with the use of quotation marks, should be entered into the chart in the chief complaint and history of present illness section(s) describing the abusive event.
- Name of investigating officer and any action taken if the police were called.
- Document every detail, even seemingly trivial ones, such as torn clothing, smeared make-up, broken fingernails, scratches, and bruises.
- Include names of all personnel who examined or talked with the patient about the injuries or abuse in the record. All personnel who attend the patient should have collaborating notes in the chart.

4.10.1.3 Admissibility of Records

Note that records are admissible as evidence if:

- They were made during the "regular course of business"
- They were made in accordance with routinely followed procedures
- They were stored properly and access to them is limited to staff only

Even if a patient later decides that s/he does not want to pursue legal remedies, a case can still be proven by introducing the statements s/he made to people in the past about what happened. Include anything that might allow you to remember the patient's attitude, face, and experience at a later date.

4.11 Clinical Assessments and Diagnosis for the Dermatologist

In the healthcare setting, domestic violence, sexual abuse/neglect of children and elderly is diagnosed in the initial healthcare visit. Dermatology is viewed as a team member in assessment and diagnosis of abuse or neglect and is often times called upon to confirm a report by the primary care practitioner.

While primary practitioners, geriatricians, pediatricians, and family practitioners are all trained in abuse and neglect, it is often the dermatologist who makes the definitive diagnosis with skin injuries, rashes, and other indicators of abuse.

4.12 Multidisciplinary Approach

In domestic violence, abuse, and or neglect, best outcomes are reported by using a multidisciplinary approach. In building a case for domestic violence and abuse/neglect, a multidisciplinary report offers the whole picture for events occurred to the patient, and provides a timeline for outcomes from initial contact with healthcare systems through treatment and follow-up. The identification of suspected domestic violence, abuse or neglect, multidisciplinary teams, including dermatology, is often the best determiner of abuse.

Persons who have been victimized through domestic violence, abuse, or neglect often require medical care and healthcare providers are most often the initial point of contact.

References

1. United States Center for Disease Control, 2000
2. Anne L. Ganley, Susan Schechter. *Domestic Violence: A National Curriculum for Family Preservation Practitioners.* 1995:17–18
3. Federal Child Abuse Prevention and Treatment Act (CAPTA) [(42 U.S.C.A. §5106 g)], as amended by the Keeping Children and Families Safe Act of 2003
4. National Elder Abuse Incidence Study (Final Report, Sept. 1998) prepared for The Administration for Children and Families and The Administration on Aging in The U.S. Department of Health and Human Services
5. Welfare Information Gateway, 2005
6. Mental Health Psychiatric Nursing
7. Family Violence Prevention Fund
8. American Journal of Preventative Medicine, June 2004
9. UN Commission of the Status of Women, 2/28/00
10. Statistics reviewed from the Bureau of Justice Crime and Victim Summary (2000–2002) report
11. World Health Organization report on Gender Based Violence
12. Toubia N. New York, New York, Women, Ink, 1993. 48 p
13. Forbes.com issue: December 2005
14. Dermatology, Chapter 105, skin signs of Physical Abuse (McGraw Hill, Access Medicine website
15. Bureau of Justice statistics
16. Centers for Disease Control
17. Corso PS, Mercy JA, Simon TR, et al Medical costs and productivity losses due to interpersonal violence and self-directed violence. *Am J Prev Med.* 2007;32(6): 474–482
18. Family Violence Prevention Fund and Educational programs Manual for health Care Professionals

Working with Other Healthcare Providers

5

Jina P. Lewallen, Carolyn Lazaro Turturro, and Angelo Turturro

5.1 Introduction

In the treatment of dermatological problems, the multi-or interdisciplinary approach encourages each discipline to bring its own training, skills, and experience to the problem-solving and treatment options for complete care of the patient. Each member of the team has a professional interest in their patient, while working in a team environment encourages each member to bring their own skills, experience, and perspective to the table. This also gives each member the flexibility to develop a care plan that meets all of the patients needs, medical and nonmedical. The team approach can be used for problem solving and for exchange of information and ideas in caring of the patient for best outcomes.

This integrated approach to medical care, although it may appear to be a product of significant recent changes in medicine (or a result of a more social approach to medicine pioneered in the 1960s), is actually much older. Working together with other professional providers for patient care was first formalized in 1905 at Massachusetts General Hospital where there was a consideration of the whole patient and the relationship between illness and social conditions in treatment.[18]

How a multidisciplinary approach works can be illustrated by considering a scenario in the pathway of care for the patient. The patient goes to his/her primary care physician (PCP), who refers the patient to a dermatologist. The communication between these two medical professionals is a vital link to the overall care of the patient. Nursing staff, lab staff, and scheduling staff are all needed to efficiently guide the patient through the healthcare pathway. Social work staff may assist in coordinating care through resources and referrals, especially for continuance of care at home. Psychiatrists, occupational therapists, and physical therapists may be called on for collaborative and collateral consultations and parallel treatments. All of these professionals on the team play an integral part in total patient care. This is especially important for dermatological care since the skin is an external organ and what afflicts the skin is often seen by other people. Their reactions can be almost as significant to the patient as the problem itself.

Multidisciplinary and/or interdisciplinary work has proven to be most effective when team members:

- Have common goals for healthcare outcomes.
- Have professional and personal commitment to care.
- Have clarification of their role on the team.
- Have the support and respect of other team members for their contributions to the team.
- Have good communication among the team members.
- Have an environment that promotes these factors.

For teaching and training, multidisciplinary/interdisciplinary teams give students a collaborative experience and view of healthcare delivery that enhances their own discipline. Students from all areas of healthcare education programs gain collaborative and extensive knowledge and skills from each member while learning about team/group process.

J.P. Lewallen (✉)
Department of Geriatrics,
University of Arkansas for Medical Sciences,
Little Rock, AR, USA
e-mail: lewallenjinap@uams.edu

R.A. Norman (ed.), *Common Treatments in Preventive Dermatology*,
DOI 10.1007/978-0-85729-853-9_5, © Springer-Verlag London Limited 2012

5.2 The Scope and Extent of Multidisciplinary Efforts

5.2.1 Scope of Multidisciplinary Efforts

Clark et al.[4] report that the joint commission on the accreditation of healthcare organizations (JCAHO) requires evidence of disciplines working collaboratively as part of its accreditation process in hospitals, nursing homes, and clinics. Bringing together different disciplines encourages an exchange of knowledge and ideas which are applied to the care of the patient. While each discipline shares basic knowledge and values (ethics) on patient care, each discipline also brings its unique contribution to the care and treatment of the patient from its perspective field.

The need for interdisciplinary, multidisciplinary teamwork has been recognized most commonly in the field of geriatrics. This may be because of the multifocal aspects of the diseases of aging and the tendency of aging to integrate these factors over the lifetime of the patient. Some of the other areas of medical care, besides dermatology, where multidisciplinary approaches are commonplace include:

- Pediatrics
- Emergency medicine
- Oncology
- Ophthalmology, ENT
- Orthopedics

5.2.2 Multidisciplinary Efforts in Dermatological Care

For dermatological care, some of the professions and roles that collaborate with the dermatologist include

- Nursing staff, who provide triage, basic medical assessment, and disease-specific care for patients
- Laboratory staff, who conduct general medical tests and diagnostics but especially dermatological-disease-specific analyses and assessments for patient treatment (some that require special training)
- Pharmacy staff, who provide drug education and support for the patient

- Social workers, psychologists, and psychiatrists, who help with nonmedical concerns and issues for the patient during treatment by the dermatologist to address the complex issues of self-image, social response, and support for the consequences of dermal disease (e.g., psoriasis)
- Genetic counseling staff, who provide genetic testing to confirm dermatological conditions that are inherited or can be passed on to further generations, for advice and support
- Health educators, who keep patients informed about their particular dermatological conditions and treatments and, along with social services, provide support for total care
- Obstetrics and gynecology, who work with dermatology on issues of skin disorders for pregnant women and as partners in total care of the patient

One consideration that should not be overlooked is that the list of disciplines involved need not be static as the patient's condition evolves, or even the same for different dermatological problems. A key aspect of the multidisciplinary approach is that different disciplines are called in as needed.

5.2.3 Challenges for Multidisciplinary Efforts

The challenges of working in multidisciplinary care teams are universal in working in any team setting. These are varied, but include:

- Determining who will be in charge of the team. In dermatological settings, it can be the dermatologist, or the PCP, or (more problematically) both as equally in charge. Patients usually need to identify with a leader who can answer questions and provide a connection between specialties during assessment and treatment.
- Clinical protocols, which can take varied pathways from general medical protocol to more specific protocol, depending on the patient's need or medical condition. The team needs to prioritize protocol for treatment and identify who will take charge of each procedure.
- Challenges that arise when two or more team members cannot agree on treatment protocol. As we know, there are varied ways to apply caring and

treatment options. It is necessary that the team members agree on assessment, diagnosis, and treatment with the best outcomes for the patient as the common goal. When challenges arise, the team should have consensus on which is the first or the best treatment protocol for the patient. This is a special area of concern since, if this is not done, treatments by different members can be at cross-purposes with no clear way to assess whether they are working or not.

- Each team member brings their own experience, level of education, and expertise which may or may not be on the same level as other team members. Team members have the opportunity to share this knowledge and experience with other team members to enrich the experience and to achieve a more level arena in which to work.

- Each discipline has its own language and philosophy of practice, so consideration for each must be addressed and an agreed on language/philosophy needs to be adopted for best patient outcomes.

5.3 Creating and Maintaining a Multidisciplinary Team

5.3.1 Creating a Team

Creating a multidisciplinary team is bringing team members from different disciplines together with shared goals and responsibilities to the patient. Team members must be able to communicate ideas and solutions openly. All members should share responsibilities, and accountability to the care of each patient. They must be willing to respect and collaborate with each team members for the best outcomes in patient care. They must also be committed to the process of team caring.

Core members of the team must all possess basic knowledge in medical care and services for the dermatology patient. The doctor, nurse, pharmacist, lab, social services professionals must all be able to communicate their roles on the team and be able to present team decision for care to the patient and families or caregivers.

Team members must meet on a regular basis during the patient's assessment and treatment phases so they can monitor the patient's progress or address any issues or concerns that arise during treatment. Each team member should be responsible for their particular piece

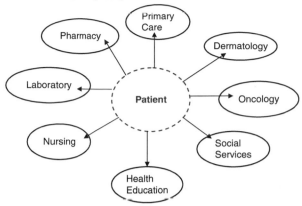

Fig. 5.1 A model of the structure of a team

of treatment and be able to present findings, address concerns, and add to the general knowledge and experience of the team.

Team members should share the lead throughout the treatment process, depending on the need of the patient during that phase of treatment in which one member has expertise. An example of this would be for a designated person to speak with the pharmacist about medication concerns, or the surgeon, if surgical intervention is part of the treatment process (Fig. 5.1).

According to the multidisciplinary team approach, the patient will have a continuum of care throughout diagnoses and treatment:

> The full continuum of care includes prevention, patient and family education, screening, staging and work-up, initial and subsequent treatment, follow-up, palliative and hospice care, and psychosocial services.[1]

With any discipline, it is important that the philosophy of treating the whole patient is in the forefront of any process. With multidisciplinary care, this may insure that the whole patient will get the continuum of care from all aspects, including medical, social, and psychological viewpoints. Including the patient and family in the team will enhance the understanding and treatment outcomes as they will be part of the process, able to access education and knowledge about their diagnosis and treatment.

5.3.2 Maintaining a Team

When a team is created it is part of a continuing commitment to multidisciplinary care to include a need for training and maintaining communication. There is a growing consensus for the need of improved communication and collaboration among healthcare providers. Clark[3] found that obstacles to effective teamwork were reported to be turf/territoriality, conflict/communication, team process, and organizational constraints with the major participant goal stated to be better collaboration at work.

5.3.2.1 Training

The development and evaluation of a teamwork model using a blend of theory and practical experience has been found to be important to the development of effective interdisciplinary strategies of patient care.[5] A training program for an interdisciplinary team might include topics focused on leadership, conflict/communication challenges, and the relationship of teamwork with quality improvement for best patient outcomes.

As an example, Clark[3] developed a leadership module that included a review of the different types of leadership styles and ways to cultivate leaders. The participants of the module discussed their observation of leadership and ways to promote leadership within healthcare teams. Teams were encouraged to gather data to evaluate both the effectiveness of the teamwork education and practice to avert backtracking to discipline- and department-specific methods when faced with financial and institutional stress. The relationship of quality improvement and teams was also presented with participants breaking-out into small groups to discuss their own experiences.[3]

5.3.2.2 Communication

Open and clear communication in multidisciplinary teams may be challenging but it is essential. Poor communication among a team of medical specialists and between family members and providers can adversely affect patient care and quality of life.[16] Patients should not have to answer the same questions over and over again to different providers. A good 20 min meeting with the family, focusing on that family and their concerns, can make admission smoother.[16] The quality of communication among a medical team has been linked to patient and family well-being in acute care settings.[2]

5.4 Special Conditions for Various Patient Groups

Multidisciplinary work with various patient groups calls on each team to customize their approach.

5.4.1 Pediatric Patients

Pediatric patients will almost always be unable to be part of the assessment and treatment plan. Parents or caregivers will usually need to assume the responsibility as a team member to advocate for their children the best course of treatment.

A special case is the occurrence of skin conditions and disorders that may appear to be normal consequences of childhood activity (like bruises and scrapes) or may be indicators or abuse or neglect. When skin conditions are present, the dermatologist can assess and detect signs of abuse and neglect vs. accidental injury, benign skin symptoms, and other skin disorders that can mimic abuse. This is particularly important as PCPs, nursing staff, social workers, therapists, and other team members may not have the expertise to differentiate between skin disorders that can mimic abuse and abuse.

This makes the inclusion of the parent as a team member a complex issue. On the one hand, the report of the dermatologist can remove the suspicion of abuse and lead to better support for the patient's parent in the team context. On the other hand, the team can be interfered with by the presence of a suspected abuser. It is important to resolve this issue before bringing the potential problem into the team. The high price to be paid when not making this determination may be the effective exclusion of the patient's advocate from the team.

5.4.2 Gerontological Patients

Many issues similar to those that arise in pediatric patients also come up in older patients, especially when the patient is incapacitated by forms of dementia. In the elderly, skin is oftentimes bruised or scratched, due to thinning skin and use of anticoagulants given to elderly for prevention of heart attack, stroke, or deep vein thrombosis (DVT). When there is a question of differentiation of diagnosis between abuse, neglect, and the by-product of medication, thin skin, or accidental injury, a dermatologist should be part of the diagnosis team. Working with other healthcare professionals can bring accurate assessments and diagnoses and enable the team to work collaboratively in treatment options or report findings as mandated by law for abuse or neglect.

A different series of issues in elderly patients are those related to the multifocal origin of problems. There is rarely, if ever, one thing wrong in the elderly. Instead there is often a constellation of events that may be involved. Leg ulcers may arise from a poor circulation, but lack of exercise (as a result of osteoarthritis), nutritional problems (from suppressed ingestion as a result of depression), and various other problems may influence disease progress. Attempts to address one problem can often set off a series of new ones. For instance, using antibiotics to fight infections often results in diarrhea. Diarrhea, in patients receiving diuretics, can easily result in hypokalemia, even in the presence of prescribed potassium. Older patients are more "fragile," i.e., with fewer reserves, so can fall into problems sooner. Considering the total patient – the hallmark of multidisciplinary efforts – becomes necessary unless the patient is to bounce from one problem to another.

5.4.3 Psychiatric Patients

These patients present with some of the same problems as children in that there are questions about who adequately represents the patient's interest on the multidisciplinary team as well as the same issues about abuse that arise in children and the elderly. However, the special needs of the psychiatric patients have stimulated interest in a new area termed psychodermatology. Focused on the boundary between psychiatry and dermatology, psychodermatology is concerned with conditions that involve an interaction between the mind and the skin.[11] Management of psychodermatologic disorders requires assessment and treatment, not only of the skin manifestation but of the psychosocial factors that may be associated with or exacerbate the condition.

Koo and Lebwohl divide psychodermatologic disorders into three broad areas. The first consists of patients with primary psychiatric disorders. These patients may present with delusions of parasitosis where they believe erroneously that they are infested with some type of organism. Other examples of primary psychiatric disorders include neurotic or psychologic excoriations, where patients self-inflict scratch marks with their own fingernails, and factitial dermatitis, where other instruments besides fingernails are used to damage skin.[11] Careful psychiatric diagnosis and treatment is of utmost important in this type of disorder and the inclusion of a psychiatrist on the multidisciplinary team is essential.

The second area includes secondary psychiatric disorders. These disorders may accompany skin conditions simply because of their visibility to other people. Conditions such as cystic acne, alopecia areata, psoriasis, hemangiomas, and Kaposi's sarcoma may be cause for psychological and social distress.[11] As cited in Koo and Lebwohl,[11] Love[12] reports that persons with skin disorders may encounter discrimination and have difficulty obtaining employment, and Ginsburg and Link[6] notes that discrimination occurs particularly when their skin disorder appears contagious. The multidisciplinary team is the perfect place to approach these problems in a holistic context, combining education, referral, counseling, and perhaps adding a legal member to the team. In addition, patients with emotional distress may be helped by the team by referral to a mental health professional or dermatological support group.[11]

The third area, and by far the most common of the psychodermatologic disorders seen in the clinic are those that can be termed psychophysiologic disorders.[11] Although discussed in context of specific disorders below, the common thread of these disorders is that these skin conditions that may be exacerbated by emotional stress. Examples include: acne, eczema, psoriasis, atopic and seborrheic dermatitis, alopecia areata, and uticaria (hives). When these skin conditions are recalcitrant to dermatologic treatment, psychosocial or occupational stress may be contributing to the disorder and warrant further investigation.[11] The treatment of chronic dermatoses may be difficult without addressing stress as an exacerbating factor. The multidisciplinary team should include members to address these areas. Stress management or relaxation techniques and exercise may be beneficial, but some issues may require counseling or therapy, antianxiety medication, or psychiatric referral.[11]

5.4.4 Other Patients

Other patients that are especially served by multidisciplinary efforts include those with language difficulties, those with problems in accessing medical care, and the under- and uninsured.

The nonmedical aspects of multidisciplinary teams may be more crucial than the medical aspects in some cases.

5.5 Special Conditions: Various Dermatological Disorders

Just as various special patient populations can influence the actions and composition of multidisciplinary groups, so can the need to address specific dermatological problems.

5.5.1 Wound Healing

Chronic wounds that are resistant to treatment add an additional risk to the patient and negatively influence their quality of life.[7] Lower extremity ulcers related to venous insufficiency are the most common type of chronic ulcer in the United States, followed by diabetic ulcers of the foot, and pressure ulcers on any body part.[13] Pain, infection, sepsis, and amputation are often associated with these ulcers.

Problem wounds had traditionally been treated by different medical specialties and healthcare workers, but over the last 20 years multidisciplinary wound healing centers have been developed in the United States as well as other countries.[7] A central clinic that uses the multidisciplinary approach to wound care can provide better patient care through more focused and efficient physician–patient encounters, a larger stock of products, and easy collaboration among specialties.[13]

Mostrow[13] described the process of developing a multidisciplinary wound clinic using the four Ps: people, places, products, and protocols. The specialties and their perspective that Mostrow[13] described include:

- Dermatologist: provides medical care of ulcers with emphasis on skin care, biopsies potential malignancies, vasculitis, and infections.
- Vascular surgeon: evaluates patients with impaired circulation for possible intervention.

- Plastic surgeon: provides special expertise in flaps and grafts, surgical debridements.
- Orthopedic surgeon: often addresses neuropathic foot ulcers, offloading pressure of ulcer and assessment of vascular supply.
- Podiatrist: provides general foot care with expertise in nails, debridement, and footwear issues.
- Nurse practitioner: runs clinic and maintains patient contact throughout week.
- Other nurses: provide patient care and education especially in relation to dressing and compression.

Gottrup et al.[7] tested the hypothesis whether "an independent, multidisciplinary wound healing center in an accepted national expert function of wound healing is the optimal way to improve prophylaxis and treatment of patients with problem wounds."

The results of the study, conducted with 23,802 patients with varying types of wounds and 1,014 patients inpatient, showed that the use of multidisciplinary teams led to improvement in healing rates and a reduction in major amputations as well as a decrease in the number of admits to the wound center.

Specifically for leg ulceration often caused by chronic venous leg insufficiency (CVI), health behaviors such as cigarette smoking and exercise are associated with circulation disorders that can influence the prognosis of CVI.[8] Heinen et al.[9] worked with a multidisciplinary project team to develop a health promotion program for patients with venous ulcers that supported adherence with compression therapy and positive lifestyle changes. The program coached patients toward adherence with compression therapy and pain management as well as leg and foot care, and targeted lifestyle behaviors of exercise, smoking, nutrition, and weight management.[9] The authors advocated development of lifestyle approaches for other patients as well.

5.5.2 Melanoma

The incidence of melanoma has risen rapidly over the past several decades. Melanoma represents the fifth most common type of cancer yet is one of the leading cancers accounting for average years of life lost per person. Often, several disciplines are needed simultaneously to optimally diagnose and treat patients with melanoma. Work-up, treatment, and follow-up recommendations may differ by physicians and healthcare providers in separate specialty settings, leading to inconsistencies in patient management and care.[10]

Specialty of the primary provider and their practice patterns have been found to influence the treatment options offered to patients with melanoma, which in turn may influence patient outcomes.[17] Evidence also suggests that multidisciplinary programs that coordinate providers and centralize care may increase patient access to comprehensive melanoma care.[17]

An example of addressing melanoma in a multidisciplinary context is provided by Johnson et al.[10] The model used was devised by the University of Michigan multidisciplinary melanoma clinic (MDMC). The process begins with the patient who has a diagnosis of melanoma. The patient goes through the process of care from the multidisciplinary view. The process is documented as:[10]

- Intake
- Direct contact via nursing staff
- Clerical for information packets and appointment
- Clinic visit, to include dermatology, surgery, social work, physical therapy, occupational therapy, etc.
- Case conference with the multidisciplinary team to assess and review plan of treatment (patient is assigned to relevant specialties with the team)
- Specialty visits, treatments
- Conference with multidisciplinary team and family for updates/changes in treatment
- Documentation management

Each patient is to be treated as "family" with each multidisciplinary member contributing their knowledge and expertise in a "turf-less" environment, dedicated to total care for the patient.

Johnson et al.[10] found that multidisciplinary melanoma care centers can optimize care of patients with melanoma and can be the most efficient plan of treatment.

5.5.3 Atopic Dermatitis

Atopic dermatitis (AD), or atopic eczema, is a common chronic, skin disorder noted by dry, itchy skin that is easily irritated. AD is the most common relapsing skin disorder in infants and children.[15] The scratching and rubbing of the itchy skin which can cause further irritation and inflammation to the skin is known as the "itch-scratch" cycle. Although stress or other emotions do not cause AD, emotions may exacerbate the "itch-scratch" cycle.[15]

It has long been recognized that treatment of AD patients has better outcomes with multidisciplinary care, especially in patients with moderate-to-severe disease.[14] The multidisciplinary team should include the PCP, nurses, nurse practitioners, physician assistants, patient advocates, social workers, and health education professionals.[14] Patient education is of special significance with emphasis on trigger avoidance, specific skin care recommendations, and follow-up.

It is also important to be clear and explicit about the use of topical medications because incorrect use of these medications is one of the primary reasons for poor treatment outcomes.[15] This is a condition where the team effort becomes a learning experience for the whole team. This is because the topical medications used are quickly evolving and what works best is currently still being worked out.

Coordinated multidisciplinary care, especially using nurse practitioners, has been successful, and results in improved care and improved satisfaction for patients, families, and healthcare providers alike.[15]

5.6 Case Study

The following case study is instructive about the multidisciplinary approach in a dermatological case.

5.6.1 Patient History

Mr. P. is an 80-year-old white male coming in with a red, scaly spot on the right side of his neck. He is seen by PCP in local hospital clinic setting.

The PCP reports to Mr. P. that the spot appears to be an irritation and gives Mr. P. a prescription for steroidal cream, to be applied twice daily.

Mr. P. returns 6 months later to report the red, scaly spot has grown and has become very itchy. The PCP reports that this is most likely a fungal infection and prescribes an antifungal ointment, twice daily.

Mr. P. sees a new PCP at a local senior health clinic and reports the spot on his neck is not getting any better. He also reports the past year's treatment with steroid and antifungal with no resolution. By this time, the spot has increased in size and remains red and inflamed. The senior health practitioner refers Mr. P. to a local dermatology clinic where he was diagnosed with squamous cell carcinoma and had surgical intervention (MONS) to remove the spot.

The follow-up below is a result of this intervention. Mr. P. was referred to the local university hospital system by the senior health clinic to review and assess Mr. P.

5.6.2 Continuation of Care of Patient Mr. P.

Mr. P. was referred to dermatology for suspected CA after squamous cell carcinoma ED and C (removed with electrodesiccation and cutterage) from face previously.

Mr. P. is an 80-year-old white male who is a new patient with history of squamous cell carcinoma ED and C from right jawline by local dermatologist, Dr. M. The patient also has history of actinic keratoses and would like to establish dermatologic care here. He denies any pain, burning, numbness, stinging, or pruritus to his recent skin cancer scars. He does have a few scaly areas to the face that are occasionally tender.

5.6.3 Physical Examination

Mr. P. is a well-developed, well-nourished white male in no acute distress. He is the primary caregiver for his 80-year-old wife who has multi-infarct dementia.

5.6.3.1 Integumentary

Scalp, face, neck, back, chest, abdomen, and bilateral upper extremities are examined. He has numerous ill-defined, scaly, erythematous papules primarily to the scalp, forehead, and the sides of his face consistent with actinic keratoses. He has a well-healed scar to the right jawline which shows no evidence of recurrence. He has a few ill-defined scaly, erythematous papules to the forearms and hands as well. He has scattered hyperpigmented stuck-on papules consistent with seborrheic keratoses. The remainder of the exam is unremarkable.

5.6.4 Assessment and Plan

1. Actinic keratoses are treated with cryosurgery for the destruction primarily to the patient's central face, on the cheeks and nose as well as arms and hands. He was given EFUDEX® to apply primarily to his forehead and scalp for the next 3 weeks, with a specific recommendation to apply it to treat the helices of his ears. Education was given on the use of EFUDEX® as well as the side effects of this medication.
2. History of squamous cell carcinoma to the right jawline, no evidence of recurrence at this time.
3. Seborrheic keratoses, benign. Will see in clinic in 3 months.

He was seen with Dr. M. (the dermatologist) with the attending physician Dr. D.

5.6.5 Dermatological Clinical Staff Call

Patient's daughter phoned stating that her father had developed a strong reaction to EFUDEX® and would like us to call patient. Patient states he has used EFUDEX® for 20 days and his face is very red and scabs "oozing" with swelling. Patient was given a Desonide by Dr. E. (an attending on call) and told to apply it to the red areas. Per Dr. M.'s review of the case, patient is to continue the Desonide to the red areas and apply Vaseline® or Aquaphor® to the areas that are crusty and oozing. Patient verbalized his understanding. He was also referred to senior health clinic.

5.6.6 Senior Health Clinic Note (Next Day)

Patient was seen in Senior Health Clinic as a walk-in due to his concern about swelling and possible infection. History of presenting illness: 80-year-old white male here today for concern about EFUDEX® treatment and redness and swelling to the face. He had been to dermatology a month ago and has been using EFUDEX® to the face for treatment of actinic keratoses. Today, he is observed having pus and drainage to the face and he is concerned about infection. He denies any fever. He states swelling is better today, but pus and drainage worse. Denies any other systemic complaints.

5.6.7 Medications

KEFLEX® 500 mg caps (cephalexin) take 1 tablet 2 times daily.

5.6.8 Dermatological Clinic Follow-Up

Mr. P. was followed up with dermatology about 2 months later with face much better and EFUDEX® and Desonide completed.

5.6.9 Multidisciplinary Assessment

Mr. P. was seen in two separate clinics, with multiple team members including.

- His PCP who gave the first referral
- Dermatology for assessment and treatment of actinic keratoses and seborrheic keratoses and history of squamous cell carcinoma
- Pharmacy which addressed medication education and information on how to use medicine and their side effects (of obvious importance in this case)
- Laboratory to review skin samples for diagnosis of squamous cell carcinoma and evaluate and monitor general health status
- Nursing staff for dermatology to take calls and review information and give advice as per doctor on treatment concerns
- Advanced practical nurse for intervention and concern for infection after treatment with other medications
- Social work for case management and support during care (again a special need in this case because much of the problem appears to have arisen from treatment)

All of these team members worked in coordination for Mr. P.'s best outcome.

5.7 Conclusion

Although generally useful, it is evident that for special patients, such as children, the elderly, and psychiatric patients, their special needs strongly support the use of multidisciplinary teams in the efficient resolution of their dermatological disorders. Also for a series of common dermatological orders, it is clear that stress, exercise, patient education, and a holistic approach to the patient is useful to improving the outcome of their treatment, sometimes dramatically. As the interface with the outside world, skin has an important role to play in how an individual feels about him/herself and how he/she relates to their social context. As such, it is not that much of a surprise that a comprehensive approach, bringing together expertise in the many areas that contribute to these complex outer and inner images, is more successful in addressing the problems that dermatological disorders bring than approaches that simply treat the skin problem like it had no effect on the life of the patient. Although multidisciplinary teams can be a complicated and cumbersome process at times, the nature of dermatological disorders is also complicated, with their effects on quality of life of equal or more concern to patients than the strictly medical problem itself.

References

1. Anon. The American Federation of Clinical Oncologic Societies access to quality cancer care: consensus statement. *J Clin Oncol.* 1998; 164:1628–1630
2. Boyle DK, Miller PA, Forbes-Thompson SA. Communications and end-of-life care in the intensive care unit: patient, family, and clinician outcomes. *Crit Care Nurs Q.* 2005; 28(4):302–316
3. Clark PG. Evaluating an interdisciplinary team training institute in geriatrics: implications for teaching teamwork theory and practice. *Educ Gerontol.* 2002;28:511–528
4. Clark PG, Leinhaus MM, Filinson R. Developing and evaluating an interdisciplinary team training program: lessons taught and lessons learned. *Educ Gerontol.* 2002; 28:491–510

5. Clark PG, Puxty J, Ross LG. Evaluating an interdisciplinary geriatric education and training institute: what can be learned by studying processes and outcomes? *Educ Gerontol*. 1997;23(7):725–744

6. Ginsburg IH, Link BG. Psychosocial consequences of rejection and stigma feelings in psoriasis patients. *Int J Dermatol*. 1993;32:587–591

7. Gottrup F, Holstein P, Jorgensen B, Lohmann M, Karlsmar T. A new concept of a multidisciplinary wound healing center and a national expert function of wound healing. *Arch Surg*. 2001;136:765–772

8. Heinen MM, van Achterberg T, op Reimer WS, et al Venous leg ulcer patients: a review of the literature on lifestyle and pain-related interventions. *J Clin Nurs*. 2004;13(3): 355–366

9. Heinen MM, Bartholomew LK, Wensing M, Kerkhof P, Achterberg T. Supporting adherence and healthy lifestyles in leg ulcer patients: Systematic development of the lively legs program for dermatology outpatient clinics. *Patient Education and Counseling*. 2006;61:279–291

10. Johnson TM, Chang A, Redman B, et al Management of melanoma with a multidisciplinary melanoma clinic model. *J Am Acad Dermatol*. 2000;42:820–826

11. Koo J, Lebwohl A. Psychodermatology: the mind and skin connection. *Am Fam Physician*. 2001;64:1873

12. Love B, Byrne C, Roberts J, Browne G, Brown B. Adult psychosocial adjustment following childhood injury: the effect of disfigurement. *J Burn Care Rehabil*. 1987;8: 280–285

13. Mostrow EN. Wound healing: a multidisciplinary approach for dermatologists. *Dermatol Clin*. 2003;21:371–387

14. Nichol NH, Boguniewicz M. Successful strategies in atopic dermatitis management. *Dermatol Nurs*. 2008;suppl:3–19

15. Nicol NH. Multidisciplinary teams are critical in the care of atopic dermatitis patients. *Medscape Dermatol*. 2005;6(2) @2005 Medscape 12/20/2005

16. Penson RT, Kyriakou H, Zuckerman D, Chabner BA, Lynch TJ Jr. Teams: communication in multidisciplinary care. *Oncologist*. 2006;11:520–526

17. Stitzenberg KB, Thomas NE, Ollila DW. Influence of provider and practice characteristics on melanoma care. *Am J Surg*. 2007;193:206–212

18. Tanaka M. Multidisciplinary team approach for elderly patients. *Geriatr Gerontol Int*. 2003;3:69–72

6

The Future of Dermatological Therapy and Preventive Dermatology

Robert A. Norman

I generally start off any of my writing in response to questions I ask myself. And I asked myself many questions when I pondered the future of the skin and prevention of skin disease. Upon reflecting on the needs of my patients and others, dozens of possibilities arose from the myriad images, smells, touch, and sounds that have filled my head from patient interactions over the years.

Although I began my inquiry with the more utilitarian potential of future skin developments, I also realized, given the enormous influence of esthetics among Homo sapiens, that the future progression will also include the "skin as entertainment" arena.

What about the skin as a vehicle for delivery of other drugs besides creams and ointments? How about providing a built-in protection for those with a heightened need for sun protection, such as those unfortunate souls with the dramatic disease xeroderma pigmentosum? Or even a safeguard for the mild, fair-haired, red-eyed lass?

What if one could change skin colors based on mood? I knew of many patients with frustrating blush disorders that had wished their state of mind was not so readily visible on their hot red skin. However, others may want a change in color, such as a military person who is trying to hide from an approaching enemy. And of course there will be those who suffer a certain ennui from their current display of tattoos, and an everchanging tableaux would offer an extensive realm of show and tell.

What will the future of dermatology be like? What will be the new detection options? What will be the new treatment options? What will be the new educational and patient teaching options? How will ethics and patient selection be challenged? How will integrative therapies and cosmetic surgeries evolve?

Skin diseases can be expensive and time-consuming and affect self-esteem, personal relationships, and careers. They also have health implications – predisposing individuals to infection, scarring, and other diseases.

As immunosuppressive and laser research are still in their infancies, the future of these fields appears boundless with new therapies constantly in development. Obviously, the continuous appearance of new treatments necessitates the regular update and revision of a physician's standard practice methods.

Dermatological concerns are among the most common consults physicians and pharmacists get if you consider hair, skin, and nails. Therapy in dermatology, particularly in the treatment of psoriasis and eczema, is changing significantly as new approaches to therapy reach the market and already-marketed products find new uses. As a result of the increased understanding of the molecular mechanisms of skin diseases, dozens of drugs are in phase II or III trials. The "survivors" in this arduous contest will reach the market in the near future.

6.1 The Genetic Century

What will be other new treatment options for diseases such as xeroderma pigmentosum? The disease, characterized by defective DNA repair, with young bearers of this autosomal recessive condition having severe solar damage and skin cancers, pigmented dry skin, and eye abnormalities, have fought an uphill battle for many years. Incorporating bacterial repair enzyme T4 endonuclease V (T4N5) into a liposomal delivery vehicle and applying it to the skin results in markedly decreased

R.A. Norman
Nova Southeastern University,
Ft. Lauderdale, FL, USA and
Private Practice, Tampa,
FL, USA
e-mail: skindrrob@aol.com

R.A. Norman (ed.), *Common Treatments in Preventive Dermatology*,
DOI 10.1007/978-0-85729-853-9_6, © Springer-Verlag London Limited 2012

skin damage. With the virtual completion of the Human Genome Project mapping of 30,000 genes, genomic maps will be available to guide the efforts to determine the genetic basis of disease. We will be able to determine response to treatment and chart a person's prognosis with greater efficiency. The twenty-first century will be the "genetic century" as we discover how the mutations bring on skin disease and the multiple mechanisms surrounding their expression.

With specific diseases such as melanoma, hope is on the horizon to replace traditional chemotherapy. Pills such as BAY 43-9006 (Sorafenib), which should reach the market within 3 years, are a new generation of "targeted" therapies that are transforming the treatment of horrible diseases such as melanoma. The pill attacks the underlying molecular mechanism and will allow cancers to be treated as a chronic disease such as high blood pressure, diabetes, or depression. Specifically, the new cancer drug attacks malignant tumors by blocking a chain reaction inside the cancer cells that allows them to multiply and attract blood vessels for growth.

6.2 New Skin

The skin is a marvel. In the best circumstances, it heals itself if broken down, repairing and restoring its former integrity. It is dour in sorrow, radiates warmth in love, and shines in tranquillity. The skin is an organ in and of itself, with its own personality, temperament, and particular eccentricities.

Its crucial body-covering role is becoming increasingly recognized, as well as the time it can use an outside boost. With almost every trauma, it rebounds, but in burn victims who have lost more than 40% of their skin surface, a temporary cover by a meshwork of donor human skin or grafts is needed. In the future, more lasting and durable skin substitutes will be needed. Likely candidates will include artificial matrices to grow skin from stem cells taken from the foreskin or umbilical cord of newborn infants. Others will use epidermal cells on an artificial dermis.

Other options are appearing, such as a three-dimensional matrix composed of a combination of human skin cells and biodegradable polymers. The bilayered matrix acts as both a foundation and environment on which the dermal cells grow and shape. The porous underlayer allows the ingrowth of human dermal cells

and the outer layer, entirely synthetic, is designed as a barrier against infection, water loss, and ultraviolet light. The human dermal cells taken from neonatal foreskin are seeded and adhere onto the polymer matrix and allowed to incubate for several weeks. The cells multiply and organize themselves into functioning tissue and can be applied to replace damaged skin.

Chemically bonding collagen taken from animal tendons with glycosaminoglycan (GAG) molecules from animal cartilage to create a simple model of the extracellular matrix also may provide a new dermis.

6.3 Teaching, Detection, Therapy, and the Modern Era

What will be the new educational options in dermatology? I discussed this with Ben Barankin, M.D. He stated:

> We will have virtual learning on the Internet with personalized medical histories and genetic tracking. As more physicians become computer and Internet savvy, and as the resources on the Internet improve, a physician will be able to sit down with the patient and their laptop to show other people with the same condition on dermatology atlas websites, as well as to recommend patient support groups, and other good resources of information. Also, physicians will be able to take pictures of the patient, and to show them what their potential scar will look like following the procedure, for those concerned with their scar appearance. The new computer systems will integrate digital photography, touch screens, voice recognition, downloads to pharmacies and HMO's to streamline the patient interactions. There will certainly be therapeutic options for those with genetic diseases. This will include most probably oral forms of medication that dermatologists and medical geneticists will collaborate on in terms of development and provision to patients. There will be further developments in the treatment of skin cancers using creams, and children will be vaccinated against a multitude of wart virus strains so as to prevent their development. As far as detection, there will be computers and robots that will do full-body scans on a semi-annual basis and be able to compare changes in moles or other concerning external and internal developments. Physicians will be there to verify these findings, biopsy as necessary, and initiate treatment.

New devices to detect skin cancer and other skin maladies include image analysis and computer-assisted diagnosis, multispectral imaging and automated diagnosis, confocal laser microscopy, optical coherence tomography, ultrasound, magnetic resonance imaging, spectrophotometric intracutaneous analysis, and artificial neural networks. Continuous research and refinement will allow improvements in detection and treatment.

Teledermatology (computer-assisted, long-distance transmission of dermatological cases) will allow detection and therapeutic suggestions to areas where hands-on dermatology is limited. Dr. Joe Kvedar of Harvard Medical School writes, "characterized as time-and place-independent care delivery, the exploding global computing network infrastructure (Internet) offers the opportunity for delivery of care anytime, anywhere. This care delivery method will enable dermatologists to offer services in a place-independent fashion and may interrupt current referral networks."[1]

Tania J. Phillips, M.D., Professor of Dermatology at the Boston University School of Medicine, stated:

> I think teledermatology will play an increasing role, physician extenders will be increasingly used, and instruments such as the dermatoscope and other in vivo imaging techniques will be used. Treatments such as the immune response modifier molecules and biologics will be increasingly used for different indications. Hopefully for wound patients there will be new, affordable cell based therapies available. For education and teaching I think that the internet and computer based learning will supplant many of our traditional methods, as they are already doing!

What else is coming up over the horizon?

Long-lasting fillers that will more permanently repair defects and make changes are being studied. The future of these skin enhancers should include a plethora of exciting new products and techniques.

Face transplants have been done; a radical procedure intended for patients with severe disfigurement. Although doctors in the past have successfully reattached faces to patients after accidents, transferring facial tissue and blood vessels from a cadaver to a new patient may become more common. Although the transplant also brings a lifetime dependence on expensive immunosuppressant drugs to block rejection of the new tissue, the operation could offer an improved future for those who suffer severe burns, cancer, or gunshot wounds. Of course, the procedure raises major moral, ethical, and psychological issues.[2]

At the Georgia institute of technology, researchers have developed micro-thin implantable films that release medication according to changes in temperature. The device will allow patients to forgo daily injections and pills including insulin, hormone therapy, chemotherapy, biologics for psoriasis and other dermatological diseases, and other treatments.[3]

Hair growth and transplantation will be safer and the individual, artificial-appearing hair plugs will be a historical reference. New and more individualized hair growth drugs will become available. Cloning of individual hair cells will allow an unlimited source of replacement hair.

Mike Morgan, M.D., provided his reflections on the "brave new world of dermatology" and changes to be expected in diagnosis:

> In the near term of the next 20 years the dermatopathologist will continue to assume the primary responsibility of diagnosis although there will be changes in who reports the diagnosis and how it is accomplished. Increasing fiscal pressures exerted by third party payers and Medicare debt will force the application of technologies such as telepathology, that were initially intended for improving medical care access, to be subverted under the pretext of cheaper medical care. Familiarity with this concept by managed-care executives and its passive approval by dermatologists will eventuate in diagnosis performed by anonymous pathologists in offshore locations as has been recently witnessed in the radiologic field. Domestically, these technologies and the applied mantra of "economies of scale" could serve as a rationalization for centralization and a monopoly of diagnostic services by well-connected individuals or singular corporate entities. Ongoing scientific discoveries and the application of nascent technologies will however eventually lead to wholesale changes in the diagnosis and management of cutaneous disorders. The dermatologist of the late twenty-first century will assume a greater degree of responsibility for diagnosis. Armed with hand-held spectrophotometric and chemical detection devices the vast majority of cutaneous neoplasms will not only be accurately identified but risk assessed in situ. Characteristic light diffraction spectra will differentially fingerprint the types of cutaneous malignancy and the application of light or sound emitting devices will precisely gauge the depth of tumor penetration. Chemical detecting devices programmed to recognize subtle changes in the metabolic by-products of cancerous cells will complement the light-emitting devices. Similarly, these devices will be relied upon to assess the extent of residual disease. Computerized algorithms that reconcile the measured variables of epidermal thickness, vascular density and depth of inflammatory infiltrate with preprogrammed archetypes will also permit the assessment and identification of many derma-toses. Such advances will undoubtedly change the role of and importance of dermatopathology in the equation of dermatologic care. As they would be relegated to the arbitration of equivocal cases or sought in the assessment of confounding data or following incomplete response to therapy.

From an ethical standpoint, Internet-based "virtual details" on new products will become more common.

Hopefully, less bias in prescribing based on personal influence from pharmaceutical companies and more objective, evidence-based data and research findings will result. Virtual details will help us to make our own decisions and not be influenced as much by the "drug reps" that wish us to sway our prescription-writing choices toward their products.[4]

The future of integrative therapies in dermatology, in particular preventive medicine, botanicals including antioxidants, hypnosis, and behavioral modification will allow new detection and treatment options. Based on research in integrative medicine, new educational and patient teaching options will be utilized in dermatology.

Future scientific discoveries may demonstrate humoral connections for many dermatologic diseases that we have long suspected to be autoimmune. Through a mixture of good clinical observation and dumb luck, we will make more connections. However, we must still discover whether these are an epiphenomena or actually a factor in disease formation. We may soon look at the age of dermatological surgery for skin cancers with a healthy nostalgia when immune therapies and vaccines replace the need for these difficult, time-consuming surgeries.

What about the future detective? We may have skin detective agencies utilizing bacteriological forensic techniques, pointing to individuals at the scene of a crime. Perhaps the characteristic microflora of a criminal suspect could be just as important to the detective as a fingerprint or other genetic markers. If an individual's microflora, established shortly after birth, remains comparatively constant throughout life, a microbial sampling of room dust, saliva, and so on, might reveal groups of identifiable organisms which would match the pattern of a suspect. The particular manner of acquisition of the many different phage-types of bacteria from mother, hospital, and early contacts could differentiate two suspects who would support different organisms. By sophisticated phage-typing methods, bacteria could be called to give evidence in court. The creation of a bio-chip that can be implanted into the skin of people to transmit their personal and medical information will be fodder for legal and scientific inquiry.

Perhaps the old adage about "what you don't see can't hurt you" applies. The huge majority or those critters that live on the skin are invisible and earn our indifference. And when it does bother us, at least we have treatments. As far as I know, we are the only species to have dermatologists, and nail salons, and beauty parlors, and a myriad of other sources to rid our body of real or perceived ailments. I am forever humbled, for along with my fellow soldiers who fight these ever-lasting skin diseases, I know we can never win the battle. However, when I think about the thousands of patients I treat with skin problems every year, I hope to provide solace from the onslaught of our own invaders. I'm glad I can provide a little help along the way and I'm looking forward to the future and what more we can offer.

Thanks to Mike Morgan, M.D.; Lisa Hutchinson, Pharm.D., MPH; Ben Barankin, M.D.; David Elpern, M.D.; and Tania Phillips, M.D. in the preparation of this chapter.

References

1. Watson AJ, Bergman H, Kvedar JC. Teledermatology. eMedicine from WebMD. Updated 27 Feb 2007. <http://wwwemedicine.com/derm/topic527.htm.>; 2009 Accessed 8.03.09
2. BBC News. "Woman has first face transplant." Available at: <http://news.bbc.co.uk/1/hi/health/4484728.stm>; 2009 Accessed 8.03.09
3. Heat-controlled Drug Implants Offer Hope for Future. Available at: <http://www.sciencedaily.com/releases/2004/09/040914092120.htm>; 2009 Accessed 8.03.09
4. Norman R. *The Woman Who Lost Her Skin and Other Dermatological Tales*. New York: Routledge; 2004

Wound Prevention

7

Cynthia A. Fleck

As the US population ages, the number of persistent and recurring wounds will continue to rise. Knowledge of key prevention practices and guidelines will help save patients from possible pain and suffering, as well as keep treatment costs to a minimum. Chronic wounds are caused by a variety of issues. Among the many factors, the aging process by itself takes its toll, predisposing the skin to wounds and other problems such as xerosis and skin tears. The clinical implications of aging are numerous and contribute greatly to the incidence and prevalence of wounds. For example, dry, inelastic skin with larger, more irregular epidermal cells leads to decreased barrier function.[1] Flattening of the dermal-epidermal junction (rete ridges) has been observed with the height of the dermal papillae declining by 55% from the third to ninth decade of life.[2] As the spaces between the well-vascularized dermis and epidermis increases, several functional changes occur:

- A 30–50% decrease in epidermal turnover rate during the 30s–80s.[1]
- Loss of sub-Q fat reduces protection from injury from pressure, shear, and friction.
- Decreased sensory perception increases risk of mechanical forces such as pressure.

A cross-sectional diagram of the changes that occur during the aging process are illustrated in Fig. 7.1.

Wound prevention in the geriatric patient therefore, requires a multifaceted approach, considering the etiology of each wound type. Within this chapter, the most prevalent wound categories will be described with practical measures for preventing these troublesome wounds, as well as other prevention topics related to wounds, such as skin care, support surfaces, and nutrition.

7.1 Venous Insufficiency Ulcers

Venous ulcers, also known as venous hypertension ulcers or venous insufficiency ulcers are caused by problems with venous blood return to the heart potentially produced by nonfunctioning or inadequate calf muscle pump, incompetent perforator valves, ineffectual valves in the vein, arteriovenous (AV) fistulas, venous obstruction, and varicose veins,[3] all leading to venous hypertension as venous blood pools in lower extremities and feet. Chronic venous disease is most likely the underlying cause in 80–95% of lower leg ulcers.[4,5] The skin is often firm, indurated and hyperpigmented, or "stained" a brown or deep color (Fig. 7.2).[6]

7.1.1 Lower Limb, Calf Pump, Maintenance Compression, ABI/TBI, ETC

Some prevention tactics that should be embraced by individuals with venous insufficiency include:

C.A. Fleck
The American Academy of Wound Management (AAWM), Washington, DC, USA and
The Association for the Advancement of Wound Care (AAWC),
St. Louis, MO, USA and
Clinical Marketing,
Medline Industries, Inc.,
St. Louis, MO, USA
e-mail: cynthiafleck@sbcglobal.net

Fig. 7.1 (**a**) Cross-section of youthful skin; (**b**) cross-section of elderly skin (Courtesy Medline Industries, Inc. Used with permission)

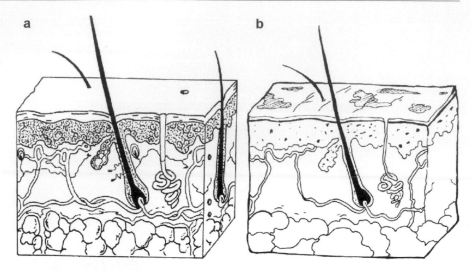

Fig. 7.1 (**a**) Cross-section of youthful skin; (**b**) cross-section of elderly skin (Courtesy Medline Industries, Inc. Used with permission)

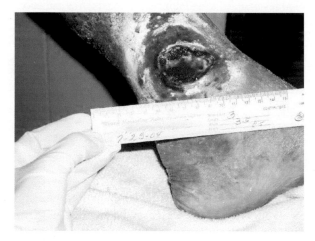

Fig. 7.2 Venous insufficiency ulcer

- Do not smoke.
- Consume adequate nutrition. Keep skin clean and well lubricated.
- Elevate the legs above the heart.
- Avoid sitting with the legs crossed.
- Avoid standing for prolonged periods of time.
- Ambulate as tolerated several times a day.
- Take medications as prescribed.
- Use compression therapy as prescribed applying every morning before rising.
- Take care of your skin.
- Follow-up with the healthcare provider.
- Elevate the foot off the bed while sleeping.
- Exercise the feet and ankles when the legs are elevated.
- Avoid the use of constrictive clothing.

Patients should undergo a lower-extremity examination, including determination of circulatory status via appropriate diagnostics (duplex imaging, Doppler, Doppler ultrasonography, air plethysmography, venography), pedal pulses, skin temperature, venous refill, color changes, skin changes (edema, hemosiderosis, venous dermatitis, atrophie blanche, varicose veins, ankle flare, scars from previous ulcers, tinea, or lipodermatosclerosis) and presence of paresthesias. A simple, noninvasive indirect method to assess arterial flow by comparing systolic blood pressure in the ankle to brachial pressure is called an ankle brachial index (ABI).[7] It is also known as the ankle brachial pressure index (ABPI), ankle/arm index (AAI), and the resting pressure index (RPT). This measurement provides the best noninvasive approximation of central systolic pressure.[8] The ABI is a screening test to identify large-vessel peripheral arterial disease by comparing systolic blood pressures in the ankle to the higher of the brachial systolic pressures. Its purpose is to detect large-vessel peripheral arterial disease in lower extremities,[9] determine adequate arterial blood flow in the lower extremities, and provide documentation of adequate arterial blood flow in lower extremities before applying compression therapy.[10]

If the ABI is higher than 1.3, indicating severe peripheral vascular disease (PVD), a toe brachial index (TBI) is recommended.[11] This is often true in diabetics or patients with renal failure where the ABI may not be properly diagnosed due to calcified vessels not allowing compression. In that case, ABI values will be false because the blood pressure will be overestimated. Both examinations compare favorably with angiographic studies in lower extremity arterial disease (LEAD) diagnosis.[12]

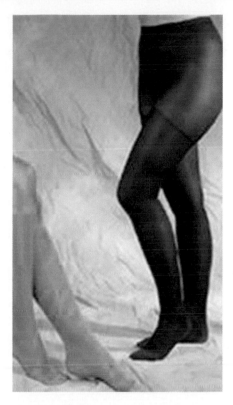

Fig. 7.3 Compression hosiery for lower extremity venous insufficiency and venous wound prevention

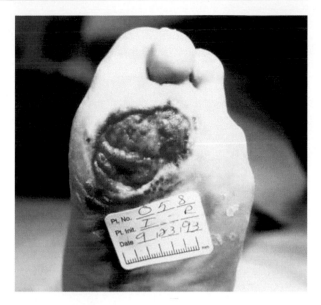

Fig. 7.4 Diabetic ulcer

Patients with untreated varicosities and/or a history of deep vein thrombosis are at higher risk for development of venous insufficiency wounds. Maintenance compression with stockings (that are replaced every 3 months to provide optimal compression) (Fig. 7.3) or other compression devices are the mainstay for prevention of venous edema and venous related wounds, which tend to recur frequently. With regard to recurrence, the evidence is insufficient to support the use of medications such as anabolic steroids[13] or the performance of vein surgery[13] to prevent these ulcers. In addition, active treatment of any varicosities should include attention to one's weight and a regular exercise program, as well as an articulated education plan that includes avoidance of leg crossing, wearing of constricting garments, etc.

Diabetic/neuropathic wounds are caused by pressure and/or trauma, secondary to peripheral neuropathy and/or arterial insufficiency and poor microvascular circulation, inadequate blood sugar control and/or lack of sensation (Fig. 7.4). Foot ulcerations are extremely common in the neuropathic patient. These ulcers often lead to complications that can result in amputation. Therefore, it is imperative that these wounds be prevented. The following measures can decrease the potential for developing a diabetic/neuropathic wound. These actions should be taught to the patient and family members to decrease the incidence of developing these wounds:

- Perform daily foot care (inspect the feet, wash and dry well between toes, wear clean socks that wick moisture away from the skin and preferably have no seams or mended areas to irritate or cause pressure).
- Prevent xerosis of the feet by applying a good-quality moisturizing cream after drying the feet. Do not apply it between the toes however, as this could increase the likelihood of fugal manifestation.
- Avoid soaking the feet.
- Avoid wearing shoes without stockings or socks, and do not wear sandals with thongs between the toes.
- Visit a healthcare professional for foot care for toenails, corns, and calluses.
- Avoid over-the-counter medications for corns and calluses, antiseptic solutions, and adhesive tape.
- Avoid crossing the legs.
- Reduce pressure on bony prominences, especially on the foot.
- Avoid temperature extremes (cold and hot).
- Avoid external heat sources, including heating pads, hot water bottles, hydrotherapy, and other hot surfaces.

- Follow-up with a healthcare provider on a routine basis. Notify the provider immediately if a sore, blister, cut, or scratch develops.
- Avoid smoking.
- Keep diabetes under control.
- Consider referral to an appropriate dietician or nutritionist.
- Be aware of poor eyesight and its affect on the overall self care of the patient.

Footwear specifics for lower extremity neuropathic disease as recommended by the Wound, Ostomy and Continence Nurses Society[14] include:

- Avoid friction from ill-fitting shoes.
- Wear well-fitting, therapeutic, customized shoes that effectively off-load problematic feet and deformities.
- See a foot wear specialist such as an orthotist or pedorthist who can choose or manufacture appropriate foot wear.
- Follow shoe design recommendations:
- Allow for 0.5 in. of space beyond the longest toe.
- Allow adequate width/depth for toe spread.
- Ensure adequate ball width.
- Check for adequate heel-to-ball fit.
- Shoes should match the shape of the foot.
- Follow shoe fitting recommendations:
- Shoes should be fitted in the afternoon when edema tends to peak.
- Patients should stand and walk when being fitted for shoes.
- Socks or stockings that would normally be worn with the shoes should be worn when fitting new shoes.
- Both feet should be measured and shoes fitted to the larger foot.
- Wearing of new shoes should be increased gradually 1–2 h at a time with a routine foot inspection to check for areas of pressure following each wearing session.
- Appropriate commercially available shoes include:
  – Made of natural materials such as leather.
  – Have cushioned outer soles and removable inner liners.
  – Have a deep toe box.
  – Secure with laces or hook-and-loop fasteners.
- Wear orthotic footwear to correct an altered gait or orthopedic deformities.
- Inspect the inside of shoes every day for foreign objects, nail points, torn linings, and rough areas.

Patients who used therapeutic footwear showed lower foot pressures as compared to those who did not. New ulcer occurrence is significantly higher in those patients who did not wear therapeutic gear.[15] Research also suggests that only 22% of individuals who own diabetic shoes wear them all day as prescribed, although most wear them periodically.[16,17]

A multidisciplinary prevention approach is recommended for persons with diabetes, insensate feet, and peripheral neuropathy.[18] Individuals at risk for foot ulceration (considering loss of protective sensation, history of previous ulceration or amputation, elevated plantar pressure, rigid foot deformity, poor diabetes control [HgA1c > 7%], diabetes of greater than 10 years duration) need to be identified early.[18]

High-risk individuals should be referred to foot care specialists for on-going preventative care and lifelong surveillance.[18] A neuropathic foot screening to identify current foot problems and initiate a prescription for appropriate prevention measures and treatment, based on risk category, should be performed at regular intervals.[19] It is recommended that a lower extremity amputation prevention program be undertaken, including annual foot screening for at-risk individuals, on-going patient education, assistance with appropriate footwear selection, patient teaching of daily foot assessment, and management of simple foot problems.[20]

7.2 Arterial and Ischemic Ulcers

LEAD is a progressive and persistent disorder affecting about 33% of US seniors (see Fig. 7.5).[21] LEAD is triggered by cholesterol deposits (atherosclerosis), PVD, and blood clotting disorders (emboli). Insufficient arterial blood supply to the lower limb leads to full or partial obstruction of the artery resulting in tissue ischemia and ultimately, necrosis.[21] Advanced age, hyperlipidemia, tobacco use, diabetes mellitus, hypertension, obesity, inactivity, and a family history of cardiovascular disease predispose one to LEAD.[22] LEAD negatively influences individuals, families, and ultimately, society. Ten to twenty-five percent of individuals with LEAD progress to critical limb ischemia within 5 years and 3–8% experience limb loss.[22] The overall price to treat lower limb ulcers is approximately $1 billion annually in the US alone, not including the countless

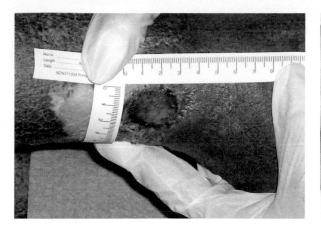

Fig. 7.5 Arterial ulcer

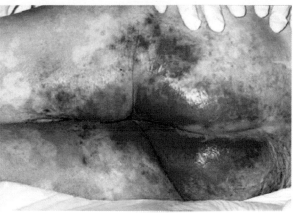

Fig. 7.6 Perineal dermatitis

lost work days. In addition, the annual cost of LEAD-induced amputations in the United States is about $5 billion.[21] Early diagnosis is often a challenge due to fewer than 50% of individuals with LEAD exhibiting typical clinical signs and symptoms connected with LEAD. Therefore, clinicians frequently use unpredictable assessment techniques for diagnosing disease.[21]

These wounds may be present in patients with diabetes and as mentioned earlier, PVD. It has been estimated that PVD affects 30% of older individuals, ages 55–74.[23] Risk factors include high blood pressure, coronary artery disease, age, diabetes, obesity, hyperlipidemia, and smoking. The patient will often complain of pain upon leg elevation and/or nocturnally, and frequently prefer to dangle their legs for optimal blood flow.[24]

Patients should be educated on life-style changes to minimize situations that cause vasoconstriction including: avoidance of smoking, exposure to cold, and wearing constricting clothing, as well as how to alleviate ischemic pain by ambulation or dangling their legs. If able, the patient with a high-risk of arterial ulcers and/or compromised arterial blood flow should be encouraged to ambulate and take part in a regular exercise program.

7.3 Perineal Dermatitis and Denudation

Perineal or "diaper" dermatitis (Fig. 7.6) is a cutaneous eruption in the diaper area caused by frequent and prolonged use of a diaper or underpad trapping urine and/or feces close to the skin. It is caused by an interaction between several factors:

- Frequent and prolonged skin wetness from occlusion and urine caught close to the skin.
- Friction by movement of the skin against skin, the diaper, the plastic leg gatherings, or the fastening tape.
- The presence of fecal enzymes that may cause cutaneous irritation coupled with bacterial or yeast growth in a dark, moist environment on inflamed, damaged skin.

Perineal dermatitis is common in infants and those adults who wear basic incontinence products that do not adequately wick away moisture.[25] If this type of dermatitis is present for longer than 3 days, there is likely to be secondary *Candida albicans* infection.[26] Generally, perineal dermatitis presents clinically as bright red, painful erythema with or without papules, erosions, scale and/or maceration, initially sparing the skin creases, on the lower abdomen, groin, perineum, buttocks, labia majora, scrotum, penis, or upper thigh.

Maintaining perineal skin integrity is one of the biggest challenges in long-term and extended-care settings, where 50–70% of patients suffer from urinary incontinence.[27] Perineal skin injury has been found in as many as one-third of hospitalized adults.[28]

Though rarely used in clinical practice, the literature describes two different assessment tools: the Perineal Dermatitis Grading Scale and the perirectal skin assessment tool (PSAT). The PSAT measures the degree of skin breakdown while the Perineal Dermatitis Grading Scale is more like a wound and skin assessment, specifically

Fig. 7.7 Perineal assessment tool (PAT)[30]

Perineal Assessment Tool
P.A.T.

Intensity of irritant Type and consistency of irritant	3 Liquid stool with or without urine	2 Soft stool with or without urine	1 Formed stool and/or urine
Duration of irritant Amount of time that skin is exposed to irritant	3 Linen/pad changes at least every 2 hours	2 Linen/pad changes at least every 4 hours	1 Linen/pad changes every 8 hours or less
Perinealskin condition Skin integrity	3 Denuded/eroded with or without dermatitis	2 Erythema/dermatitis with or without candidiasis	1 Clear and intact
Contributing factors Low albumin, antibiotics, tube feeding, or *C. Difficile* infection, other	3 3 or more contributing factors	2 2 contributing factors	1 0-1 contributing factor

- Score of 4-6 on the PAT scale is considered "low" risk
- Score of 7-12 is considered "high" risk.

targeting location of dermatitis, skin color and integrity, amount of skin involvement, and symptoms, such as pain. The scale also includes an area for a brief description of the skin assessment or the patient's symptoms.[29]

A validated tool developed by Nix can be used to assess risk for perineal skin damage[30] The perineal assessment tool (PAT) is an instrument that identifies four determinants of perineal skin breakdown: duration of irritant, intensity and type of irritant, perineal skin condition, and contributing factors causing diarrhea. Each subscale reflects degrees of risk factors. All subscales are rated from one (least risk) to three (most risk). Each rating has a descriptor and a description of each level of the scale. Total scores can range from 4 (least risk) to 12 (most risk). A score between four and six on the PAT scale is considered a low risk, and a score between 7 and 12 is considered a high risk (Fig. 7.7).[30] This tool may be added to the assessment, along with the Braden Risk Assessment Score (Fig. 7.8).

The Wound, Ostomy and Continence Nurses Society guidelines for prevention and management of pressure ulcers offers these interventions for preventing perineal dermatitis:

- Establish a bowel and bladder program for patients with incontinence.
- Avoid excess friction on the skin.
- Cleanse skin gently at each time of soiling with pH-balanced cleansers.
- Use incontinent skin barriers as needed to protect and maintain intact skin.

- Select underpads, diapers, or briefs that are absorbent to wick incontinence moisture away from the skin.
- Consider using pouching system or collection device.[31]

The use of absorptive and/or occlusive devices has been identified as a large contributor to the problem of incontinence-associated dermatitis, leading to wounds. Prolonged occlusion of the skin under an absorptive incontinent product for 5 days has been shown to cause an increased sweat production and compromised barrier function, resulting in increased transepidermal water loss (TEWL), CO_2 emission, and pH; microflora of the skin undergoes a marked increase in coagulase-negative staphylococcus.[32]

Novel disposable underpads that allow air flow and offer advanced polymer technology provide super absorbing capacity (absorbing power of three or more pads) while locking fluid deep within the pad, keeping the patient's skin dry for better odor control and skin care (Fig. 7.9). In addition, the underpads provide a healthier skin environment, allowing air flow while acting as a barrier to moisture. They also lower overall costs (reducing the need multiple pads, reusable pads and draw sheets) and make for easier care, as they may be used on regular or low-air-loss beds.

Denudation is a form of partial thickness injury related to friction and shearing forces and chemical and enzyme irritation from incontinence.[33]

BRADEN SCALE FOR PREDICTING PRESSURE SORE RISK

Patient's Name _____   Evaluator's Name _____   Date of Assessment

SENSORY PERCEPTION ability to respond meaningfully to pressure-related discomfort	**1. Completely Limited** Unresponsive (does not moan, flinch, or grasp) to painful stimuli, due to diminished level of consciousness or sedation. OR limited ability to feel pain over most of body	**2. Very Limited** Responds only to painful stimuli. Cannot communicate discomfort except by moaning or restlessness OR has a sensory impairment which limits the ability to feel pain or discomfort over ½ of body.	**3. Slightly Limited** Responds to verbal commands, but cannot always communicate discomfort or the need to be turned. OR has some sensory impairment which limits ability to feel pain or discomfort in 1 or 2 extremities.	**4. No Impairment** Responds to verbal commands. Has no sensory deficit which would limit ability to feel or voice pain or discomfort.
MOISTURE degree to which skin is exposed to moisture	**1. Constantly Moist** Skin is kept moist almost constantly by perspiration, urine, etc. Dampness is detected every time patient is moved or turned.	**2. Very Moist** Skin is often, but not always moist. Linen must be changed at least once a shift.	**3. Occasionally Moist:** Skin is occasionally moist, requiring an extra linen change approximately once a day.	**4. Rarely Moist** Skin is usually dry, linen only requires changing at routine intervals.
ACTIVITY degree of physical activity	**1. Bedfast** Confined to bed.	**2. Chairfast** Ability to walk severely limited or non-existent. Cannot bear own weight and/or must be assisted into chair or wheelchair.	**3. Walks Occasionally** Walks occasionally during day, but for very short distances, with or without assistance. Spends majority of each shift in bed or chair	**4. Walks Frequently** Walks outside room at least twice a day and inside room at least once every two hours during waking hours
MOBILITY ability to change and control body position	**1. Completely Immobile** Does not make even slight changes in body or extremity position without assistance	**2. Very Limited** Makes occasional slight changes in body or extremity position but unable to make frequent or significant changes independently.	**3. Slightly Limited** Makes frequent though slight changes in body or extremity position independently.	**4. No Limitation** Makes major and frequent changes in position without assistance.
NUTRITION <u>usual</u> food intake pattern	**1. Very Poor** Never eats a complete meal. Rarely eats more than $\frac{1}{3}$ of any food offered. Eats 2 servings or less of protein (meat or dairy products) per day. Takes fluids poorly. Does not take a liquid dietary supplement OR is NPO and/or maintained on clear liquids or IV's for more than 5 days.	**2. Probably Inadequate** Rarely eats a complete meal and generally eats only about ½ of any food offered. Protein intake includes only 3 servings of meat or dairy products per day. Occasionally will take a dietary supplement. OR receives less than optimum amount of liquid diet or tube feeding	**3. Adequate** Eats over half of most meals. Eats a total of 4 servings of protein (meat, dairy products per day. Occasionally will refuse a meal, but will usually take a supplement when offered OR is on a tube feeding or TPN regimen which probably meets most of nutritional needs	**4. Excellent** Eats most of every meal. Never refuses a meal. Usually eats a total of 4 or more servings of meat and dairy products. Occasionally eats between meals. Does not require supplementation.
FRICTION & SHEAR	**1. Problem** Requires moderate to maximum assistance in moving. Complete lifting without sliding against sheets is impossible. Frequently slides down in bed or chair, requiring frequent repositioning with maximum assistance. Spasticity, contractures or agitation leads to almost constant friction	**2. Potential Problem** Moves feebly or requires minimum assistance. During a move skin probably slides to some extent against sheets, chair, restraints or other devices. Maintains relatively good position in chair or bed most of the time but occasionally slides down	**3. No Apparent Problem** Moves in bed and in chair independently and has sufficient muscle strength to lift up completely during move. Maintains good position in bed or chair.	

© Copyright Barbara Braden and Nancy Bergstrom, 1988 All rights reserved   Total Score

Fig. 7.8 Braden risk assessment score (Copyright Barbara Braden. Used with permission)

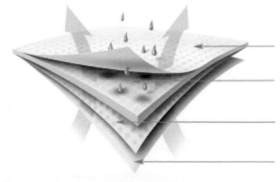

Fig. 7.9 Super-absorbent polymer underpad (Courtesy Medline Industries, Inc. Used with permission)

soft, non-woven topsheet
Soft against skin for increased comfort

Advanced SuperCare absorbent sheet
Thermo-bonded to provide pad integrity and exceptional skin dryness

AquaShield Film
Traps moisture, providing leakage protection

Innovative Backsheet
Air permeability means skin comfort

7.4 Maintaining Skin's Integrity

Skin care is a four-pronged approach with cleansing, moisturizing, protecting, and now nourishing being the key steps. The largest organ of the body, the integument, receives one third of the human body's cardiac output, feeding and nourishing it from the inside.[34] Nutrition and antioxidant protection can also take place endermically with the advent of advanced skin care products. See Table 7.1 for the hierarchy or generations of available skin care products.

7.4.1 Cleansing

Cleanser technology has come a long way from merely cleansing for the removal of sebum, soil, dirt, and bacteria to providing mildness, moisture, and now nourishment to the skin in addition to cleaning it. Harsh soaps and surfactants in cleansers can cause damage to skin proteins and lipids, inflammation and swelling of the stratum corneum, and alter lipid rigidity. This leads to tightness, dryness, barrier damage, irritation, pH disruption, increased water loss or dehydration of the skin, and itching.[35] Shocking as it may seem, soaps touted as "natural" and "safe" often have the highest and, therefore, most damaging pH. For instance, Ivory soap has a pH of 10.5 and Dial measures in at 10.0. This simple pH study looked at products commonly used in nursing homes.[36]

In order for cleansers to provide skin care benefits, they must first minimize the damage of surfactants to skin proteins and lipids. This can be accomplished by using the least harmful surfactants or, better yet, phospholipids to clean. Phospholipids are ingredients derived from selected vegetable oils that can bind both water and fat, providing excellent cleansing and conditioning properties and incredible after-feel due to their mildness. They contain naturally occurring polyunsaturated fatty acids (PUFAs), which can contribute to the activation of cellular metabolism. They are superior cleansers that do not strip, dehydrate, or inflame the epidermis. Cleansers must secondly deposit and deliver beneficial agents, such as occlusive skin lipids, humectants, amino acids, and vitamins, under wash conditions to improve skin hydration as well as mechanical and visual properties.

Soap and surfactant detergent-type cleansers can be damaging and abusive to patients' skin. Soap strips the skin of cell-binding lipids and ceramides and makes it much more vulnerable to assaults of daily living, such as skin tears. Sodium lauryl sulfate, ammonium laureth sulfate, and sodium laureth sulfate are associated with irritation and stripping skin lipids, especially when left on the skin in the "no-rinse" products. Repeated surfactant use leads to increased skin dehydration and potential damage. Another caveat to consider is to customize bathing according to patient needs. Daily baths with a bath basin and bar of high alkaline soap can be extremely detrimental to the integument.

7.4.2 Hydration

The epidermis contains lipids that play a vital role in maintaining healthy skin and regulating moisture loss. With age, the use of detergents and damage, such as burns or wounds, cause the skin to lose some or all of its ability to retain moisture. Skin becomes dry and with this dryness comes skin breakdown.

Skin needs to be protected from the environment to reduce the effects of aging. To do so, the use of skin moisturizers and protectants is beneficial. Moisturizers are complex formulations designed to maintain skin flexibility, smoothness, and barrier integrity while maintaining the water content of the skin between 10% and 30%. For skin to appear and function normally, the water content of the stratum corneum must be at least 10%. Cells are composed of 70% water. Since the skin is made up of cells, maintaining a high level of moisture in the skin is necessary. Skin that is water deficient, such as thickened skin over the heels, is often rough to the touch and fissures easily. There are two means by which to moisturize the skin. One way is to add back moisture to the skin. The other way is to block or inhibit TEWL.

Moisture is mandatory for an organ that is in constant motion. Skin hydration is important to maintain an intact barrier protection. The application of topical moisturizing and protectant products, coupled with the use of surfactant-free cleansers, helps reduce dryness and stop TEWL. In order for moisturizers to work, they must be coupled with moisture in the form of water. It either comes from the dermis

Table 7.1 Hierarchy of skin care products

Product category	First-generation products	Second-generation products	Third-generation products
Cleansers	Soaps – oldest amphiphilic cleaning agent, highly alkaline. Examples include sodium cocoyl, sodium tallowate, sodium sterate, sodium dodycelbenzensulfoate, sodium cocoate, sodium palmitate, etc.	Surfactants – synthetic detergents such as sodium lauryl sulfate, tea lauryl sulfate, cocoam-phocarboxyglaycinate, disodium oleamido mea sulfosuccinate, sodium laureth sulfate, ammonium laureth sulfate, etc.	Phospholipids – mimic the body's natural lipid requirements, ingredients derived from selected vegetable oils that can bind both water and fat providing excellent cleansing and conditioning without stripping or drying. Examples include: cocamidoproryl PG-dimonium phosphate, linoleamidopropyl PG>dimonium chloride phosphate dimethicone, disodium lauroamphodiacetate
Moisturizers emollients humectants	Lotions, creams and ointments containing lanolin, glycerin, mineral oil, propylene glycol, petrolatum, cocoa butter, paraffin, etc.	Lotions, creams and ointments containing first-generation ingredients plus ingredients such as carbohydrates like aloevera, vitamins like retinyl palmitate (vitamin A), ergocalcifrol (vitamin D), glycosaminoglycans such as hyaluronic acid, polyhydroxy hydroxy acids, urea, etc.	Lotions, creams and ointments containing first- and second-generation ingredients plus nutritive ingredients such as amino acids, vitamins and cofactors, high-quality oils and lipids such as shea butter or grape seed oil, antioxidants such as hydroxytyrosol, advanced silicones and methylsulfonylmethane
Protectants and barriers	Creams and ointments containing petrolatum, octyl hydroxysterate, etc.	Creams and ointments containing dimethicone, allantoin, zinc oxide, calamine, karaya gum, etc.	Creams and ointments containing first- and second-generation ingredients plus nutritive ingredients such as amino acids, vitamins and cofactors, high-quality oils and lipids such as shea butter or grape seed oil, antioxidants such as hydroxytyrosol, advanced silicones and methylsulfonylmethane

Copyright Cynthia A. Fleck®

(internally) or externally applied water, such as immediately following a bath or shower. The National Eczema Association for Science and Education recommends sealing in skin's moisture with a high-quality moisturizer within 3 min of showering or bathing.

7.4.2.1 Xerosis

Xerosis is dry skin that appears when there is dehydration of the stratum corneum and is one of the most common skin conditions to affect the elderly (Fig. 7.10).[37] It is most common in the aged who have decreased epidermal free-fatty acids, compared to younger skin. Xerotic skin additionally has a reduced amino acid content.[38] The patient will usually complain of dryness and itching. The condition is more prevalent in the lower legs and feet but can occur anywhere on the body. It also tends to exacerbate in winter months, and in cold and dry climates or low humidity conditions.

Moisturizers are primarily intended to help the skin to function properly in conditions where temperature and humidity are low and mimic the role of naturally occurring epidermal lipids. They are sold as creams, lotions, and in some cases serums. Lotions are the lightest and provide less protection.

The most important moisturizer, and really the only true moisturizer, is water. To maintain the water content of the skin, we can use occlusive ingredients to keep the moisture from evaporating, such as petrolatum or mineral oil, or apply water to the skin and bind it with humectants (e.g., glycerin, hyaluronic acid, chitosan, beta glucan 1–3), emollients (e.g., shea butter, avocado butter, cocoa butter), or nonocclusive ingredients, such as natural oils and silicones. One caveat is that mineral oil and petrolatum are hydrocarbons and

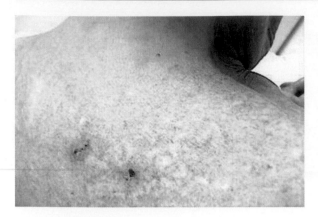

Fig. 7.10 Xerosis or dry skin with typical flaky or scaly, almost transparent appearance

do not contribute to lipid replacement. Better choices include high-quality oils like borage oil, olive oil, and rose hip seed oil.

7.4.3 Skin Protectants

When the skin needs extra protection from incontinence, periwound maceration, wound, stoma, fistula, or access site drainage or leaking, partial-thickness wounds, and denudation, barriers provide the answers. Since incontinence affects 13 million Americans or about 10%–35% of adults and at least half of the 1.5 million nursing home residents,[39] incontinent dermatitis is a common skin dilemma that often results when urine comes in contact with dry, cracked skin. It provides an excellent environment for the growth of bacteria, resulting in the production of ammonia. Ammonia increases the pH of the skin, reducing the acid mantle's protective capacity as a bacterial barrier subsequently presenting the opportunity for chemical irritation by urine, feces, and excess moisture leading to skin breakdown.[27]

Protectants or barriers provide a physical barrier between the skin and caustic bodily fluids. Ointments and creams that contain petrolatum are inexpensive and readily accessible but need to be applied frequently as they melt off and wash away quickly. They can also inhibit the absorbency of briefs, under pads, and dressings. An example is A and D Ointment. Products containing zinc oxide stay on the skin longer, providing better protection. They are thicker and allow the caregiver to simply "fill in the blanks" when reapplying after cleansing.

Dimethicone and other silicones provide sophisticated additions in many skin protectants. These ingredients provide long-lasting protection, remaining on the skin through multiple washings or cleansings. The percentage of dimethicone cannot be judged by itself since combinations of various silicones can offer better protection than just a high percentage of dimethicone alone.

7.4.4 Skin Nutrition

Maintaining healthy skin is vital to a person's overall health. As we age, the skin, like other organs in the body, begins to function less effectively, and therefore, special care is required. The use of advanced cleansers that are gentle and do not strip the skin and moisturizers and protectants to defend the skin from dryness and TEWL is essential. The replacement of soaps with cleansing lotions and surfactant-free products that protect skin lipids and aid in skin integrity is also vital.

There is a new generation of skin care products that do more than clean, protect, and moisturize. These advanced skin care products can actually nourish the skin by providing vital amino acids, vitamins, lipids, and antioxidants that were developed to protect skin from breakdown and to minimize the risk of dryness, decreased skin integrity, and invasion of pathogens. The products also bring nutrients to the skin that help restore its protective acid mantle, help reestablish collagen, and help defend against free radical damage while protecting from stinging and pain. In addition, they have been shown to decrease the prevalence of pressure ulcers and skin tears.[40] One retrospective, longitudinal study studied the changes in pressure ulcer prevalence rates and the economic effect of introducing a silicone-based dermal nourishing emollient regimen into an existing pressure ulcer protocol.[41] The results showed a decrease from 17% incidence rate down to 0% and an average cost savings of $6,677 per patient. Think of these third-generation advanced skin care products as a form of "corneotherapy," feeding and nourishing the stratum corneum.

Key ingredients and nutrients can be applied and absorbed via the skin to deliver nourishment and provide healing and health to this vulnerable organ. This is termed endermic nutrition. Enhancing the skin with the topical application of amino acids, antioxidants, and lipids may be the only external way to improve the health of this vital organ. Nutrients enter the epidermis from the dermis or the stratum corneum. Advanced skin care products truly address the needs of the cells, providing the proper nutrients in the correct forms for the skin to assimilate them, helping protect the cells against free radical damage while supplying amino acids that are the main building blocks of collagen.

7.5 Pressure Ulcers

Pressure ulcers are one of the largest dilemmas facing long-term care providers and clinicians who care for geriatric patients. Two thirds of pressure sores occur in patients older than 70 years of age.[42] Pressure ulcer prevalence is estimated to be around 15% in acute care, up to 28% in long-term care and up to 29% in home care.[43] Pressure ulcers account for $2.2–3.6 billion/year in expenditures,[44] can cost up to $70,000 to treat,[45] and kill 60,000 people in the US every year.[46] Patients inclined to pressure ulcers are at higher risk of morbidity and mortality, with infection, osteomyelitis, and sepsis being the most common major complications.

Pressure ulcers are any lesions caused by unrelieved pressure resulting in damage of underlying tissue.[47]

Pressure ulcers have affected us throughout the ages. Yet, dealing with the general management of pressure ulcers has only just begun to gain notoriety among national and worldwide healthcare concerns. In spite of present attention and development in the areas of medicine, surgery, nursing care, physical therapy, and self-care education, pressure ulcers continue to be a major source of morbidity and mortality. This is especially true for our elders and for those with impaired sensation and prolonged immobility.[48]

It is theorized that pressure ulcers are caused by localized pressure or shear forces that lead to ischemia and cell death, thus causing skin and tissue breakdown (Fig. 7.11). Pressure is equal to force, divided by area. So the greater the surface area of the load, the less pressure exerted. For instance, a sitting individual is at higher risk of developing a pressure ulcer than a person who is lying supine. Kosiak proved that tissue compression and ischemia can lead to tissue destruction and pressure ulcer formation. He also showed that the amount of pressure and the duration of the pressure are inversely proportional.[49] For instance, low amounts of pressure over longer periods of time can be just as detrimental as high pressure for shorter times (Fig. 7.12).[50]

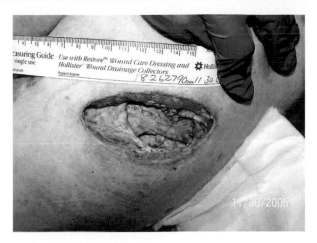

Fig. 7.11 Pressure ulcer

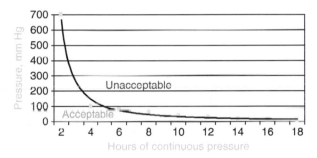

Fig. 7.12 Guidelines for sitting duration. Maximum suggested pressure/time application over bony prominences[50]

7.5.1 Causes

Although prolonged, uninterrupted pressure is the main cause of pressure ulcers, impaired mobility is probably the most common reason patients are exposed to unrelieved pressure. This is common in those who are neurologically impaired, heavily sedated or anesthetized, restrained, demented, or those suffering traumatic injury such as a pelvic or femur fracture. These patients are incapable of assuming the responsibility of altering their position to relieve pressure. Moreover, this immobility, if prolonged, leads to muscle and soft tissue atrophy, decreasing the bulk over which bony prominences are supported, further increasing the risk of developing a pressure ulcer.

7.5.2 Heel Pressure Ulcers

The heel presents a problematic source of pressure due to its bony prominence, especially in the recumbent individual. Care should be taken to mobilize the immobile, providing good skin care and off-loading with pressure relief equipment, to the vulnerable heel area. The heel is one of the most difficult anatomical areas to address by prevention products.[51] Studies have demonstrated that support surface, including special beds, mattresses, and overlays, do not provide complete pressure relief in the heel region.[52] Be aware of anti-embolism stockings, TED hose, and compression devices as they can camouflage the heels and preclude thorough assessment.

Floating the heels is recommended by many experts as well as prevention guidelines as the only viable method to completely alleviate heel pressure and prevent ulcers.[53]

7.5.3 Prevention Basics

Healthy individuals with normal sensation, mobility, and mental faculty usually do not succumb to pressure ulcers. Feedback, both conscious and unconscious, from the areas of compression leads us to change our position. We constantly make micro-movements to compensate. This shifts the pressure from one area to another prior to any irreversible ischemic damage to the tissues. Weight shifting for insensate individuals or those with poor mobility should take place every 15 min in the seated person and at least every 2 h in the recumbent individual.[54–56]

Pressure ulcer prevention encompasses alleviating the possible causative factors. If we consider that lack of viable blood flow to the tissue is the main cause of pressure ulcers, we can further classify that damage into pressure, shear, friction, moisture and heat and thus, better support the host. We can also prevent pressure ulcers by managing the following negative effects. These prevention recommendations are adapted from the 1992 agency for healthcare policy and research (AHCPR), now the Agency for Healthcare Policy and Research (AHRQ) clinical practice guidelines[53] and the Wound Ostomy and Continence Nurse Association's 2003 Guidelines for Prevention and Management of Pressure Ulcers.[57]

7.5.3.1 Pressure

- Pressure can be lessened by establishing a patient turning schedule that can be documented. The standard of care for turning and repositioning is every 2 h in the recumbent individual and every 15 min in the seated person.
- Use the 30° lateral position in a supine patient instead of placing a patient side lying at 90°. This dramatically decreases the peak pressure caused by the greater trochanter.
- Implement an appropriate pressure-redistribution support surface to both the seated and recumbent surfaces that the patient's body contacts at the first sign of risk.
- For cushioning a seated client, avoid the use of invalid rings, "donuts", rubber rings or any technology that has a "cut-out" since this can actually increase pressure, especially over bony prominences.
- Limit the time that the patient spends on the commode or bedpan.
- Off-load the heels with a pillow, heel protection device or wedge.

7.5.3.2 Shear

- Limit the elevation of the head of the bed to 30° or less.
- Use draw sheets to turn and reposition patients.
- Use the bed's side rails and consider adding a trapeze to the bed frame to optimize mobility and decrease shear forces.
- Never perform massage over bony prominences that have been compressed. This can cause tissue damage, although there is conflicting information in the literature.[58]

7.5.3.3 Miscellaneous

- Apply high-quality moisturizers to the skin to increase the water content and thus pliability and strength. Apply moisturizers anytime water comes in contact with the skin, especially after the bath or shower. Look for products that allow the skin to breath while decreasing excessive transepidermal water loss (e-TEWL).
- Use a skin prepping solution or sealant before using tape on a patient's skin.
- Teach the patient and care givers to visually inspect the skin daily for early detection.
- Encourage proper hydration and nutrition.
- Institute an active or passive range-of-motion routine.

- Calculate a risk assessment score on every patient to identify those at high risk for development of pressure ulcers (see risk assessment, Braden Scale).
- Apply transparent dressings or skin sealants to protect the epidermis.

7.5.3.4 Moisture

- Protect the skin from body fluids and drainage by absorption.
- Decrease baths and address a patient's need for skin cleansing individually and by body region.
- Use moisturizing, soap-free cleansers with a neutral or slightly acidic pH.
- Apply barrier creams that remain in contact with the skin despite cleaning to offer protection from incontinence episodes. Good examples of ingredients include zinc oxide, dimethicone, and other high-quality silicones. Products containing petrolatum-based protectants should be avoided since they protect for a very short time and do not remain in contact with the skin.
- Institute a bowel and bladder program that is customized to each resident and can be documented.
- Consider the use of some of the newer high-tech polymer-based incontinent products (briefs, pad, etc.) and customize to each resident's needs.

7.5.3.5 Seated Dependent

- Avoid uninterrupted sitting.
- Teach the patient to perform a weight shift (stand up with assist, push-up, bend at the waist, or shift from side to side) every 15 min.
- If the patient is not able to perform an independent weight shift, they should be repositioned or put back to bed once per hour.
- Utilize a high-quality pressure redistribution cushion (high-density foam, air or viscous gel) for all seated dependent individuals.

Recently, the New Jersey Hospital Association Collaborative achieved a 70% reduction in the incidence of pressure ulcers in 2 years,[59] from 18% down to 5%. They accomplished this by focusing on prevention, developing, and delivering 2 day sharing and learning sessions and continuation of best practice.

7.5.4 Support Surfaces

In the pursuit of prevention and management of skin and tissue breakdown, support surface selection remains an important decision for the clinician. Pressure ulcers are caused by a myriad of intrinsic and extrinsic factors. Support surfaces can have significant influence over extrinsic factors such as pressure, shear, friction, moisture, and temperature.[60] These factors directly impact deformation of the soft tissue, blood flow, tissue ischemia and necrosis, and pressure ulcer development, especially in the immobile patient. The manner by which support surfaces manage these extrinsic factors can be used by clinicians as they select support surfaces for their patients.

Support surfaces are specialized devices for pressure redistribution designed for management of tissue loads, microclimate, and/or other therapeutic functions as adjunctive devices to pressure ulcer prevention.

External pressure, especially over the bony prominences, has been identified as the major etiology in pressure ulcer development. Additional associated origins consist of the degree of shear and friction forces and the further effects of temperature and moisture. All of these factors can be affected by, and are correlated to, the characteristics of the support surface selected for an individual.

Clinicians typically use the term "pressure" to reflect normal pressure or interface pressure – the force per unit area that acts perpendicular to the tissue. The forces that result in normal pressure on the tissues are typically due to gravity; body weight is resting on the supporting surface. With respect to support surfaces, this normal loading may be the most significant, but it is not the only force that impacts tissue integrity.

Various clinical strategies exist to manage these extrinsic factors, especially for patients exhibiting the two greatest risk factors for pressure ulcers, diminished mobility, and/or lack of sensation. Turning and repositioning are the most effective ways to counteract impaired mobility. However, the accepted protocol of turning and repositioning a patient every 2 h may not be enough.[61] An individualized care plan must be developed that includes support surfaces as integral components to prevention and management of pressure ulcers.

Support surfaces choice and selection is one of many important decisions the clinician and team must assess, plan, implement, evaluate, and discuss for both prevention and treatment of pressure ulcers.

7.6 Skin Tears

It is important to mention skin tears, traumatic sores that tend to occur to some of the same individuals as pressure ulcers (Fig. 7.13). As the skin ages, the basement membrane (junction between the epidermis and the dermis) flattens, making it "loose," thus more prone to traumatic injury and unintentional separation, in essence, a skin tear. The anatomy of aging skin makes skin tears nearly inevitable in the elderly. In addition, harsh soaps and surfactant cleansers as well as nonnutritional moisturizers and protectants containing hydrocarbons such as petroleum and mineral oil, which do not contribute to lipid replacement, further add to the skin's vulnerability. Choosing a skin care regime that replaces soap and harsh surfactant cleansers (detergent type) with pH balanced mild cleansers and phospholipids cleansers can decrease the incidence of skin tears, additionally providing overall cost savings and comfort.

7.7 Nutrition

By far, one of the most incriminating intrinsic risk factors for the development of pressure ulcers as well as other wounds is malnutrition. Many studies cite a strong link between deteriorating nutritional status and the development and healing of chronic, nonhealing wounds such as pressure ulcers.[62–64] Up to 85% of residents in nursing homes suffer from malnutrition.[65] It is no wonder that this group of individuals is also at highest risk for the development of pressure ulcers.

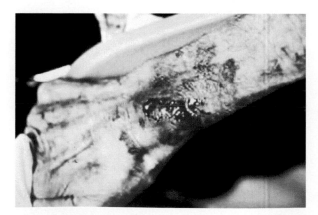

Fig. 7.13 Skin tear

A nutritional assessment can help the provider identify whether a patient has nutritional risk factors for impaired wound healing. When is a nutritional assessment indicated? There are many "red flags" to alert the provider to potential risk. An obvious one is involuntary weight loss and/or a change in the individual's appetite. Some not so apparent indicators may include impaired cognitive patterns, altered communication/hearing/vision, impaired mood/behavior, and diminished physical and functional capabilities. A Braden scale risk-assessment score below the threshold of 18 in older populations can indicate risk for development of pressure ulcers. This is an assessment that is most likely already being performed and can serve as an early warning to initiate further nutritional investigation.

A nutritional assessment investigates four basic categories: anthropometric information, biochemical data, clinical facts, and dietary history[66], and should be conducted by a registered dietician on every at-risk individual.

7.7.1 Biochemical Data

Biochemical data includes laboratory tests, such as serum albumin, serum prealbumin, serum transferrin, total lymphocyte count (TLC), and nitrogen balance.

Serum albumin is the major circulating plasma protein synthesized by the liver. It is an inexpensive blood test and common indicator of the resident's protein stores. Its half life (how long it will take before we see decreases in lab data) is about 3 weeks, so the blood you draw from your resident today will indicate their protein stores from 3 weeks ago. Mild depletion is considered 3.5 g/100 mL. Serum albumin below 3.0 g/dL (hypoalbuminemia) is associated with tissue edema, which further increases risk of pressure ulcers. Serum albumin levels are often used as an indicator of overall nutrition. Low serum albumin increases risk of infection, morbidity, and mortality. It impairs or prevents wound healing and decreases wound tensile strength.

Serum prealbumin is a more sensitive indicator of visceral protein status in acute stages of malnutrition. Its half life is only 2–3 days and can be helpful to evaluate the adequacy of nutritional therapy. Mild depletion is <15 mg/dL. Severe depletion is <5 mg/dL. If the resident has chronic renal failure, prealbumin may be falsely elevated, since it is eliminated in the kidneys.

Serum transferrin has a half life of a little over a week and is an indicator of protein stores as well. A level below 200 mg/dL is considered low. This blood test may not be useful in the presence of liver disease or estrogen use, since transferrin levels will be abnormally high. Also of note, liver disease, burns, cortisone or testosterone therapy, and chronic infection can lower serum transferrin levels.

TLC reflects the visceral (contained in the body's organs) protein stores of the body and immunity. TLC is more useful as a screening parameter in noncritical individuals. A TLC below 2,000 cells/mm^3 indicates an impaired immune system.

Nitrogen balance is also useful for assessment of protein requirements, since protein is 16% nitrogen. Nitrogen balance is the difference between nitrogen intake and output. It helps determine needs for protein maintenance and anabolism. Accurate measurements of food and fluid intake over a 24-h period and a 24-h continuous urine sample are needed. Nitrogen balance results can be questionable in the presence of renal disease.

7.7.2 Vitamins and Minerals

Many registered dietitians include multivitamin/mineral supplements as part of their preventative protocol for residents at high risk for ulcers or with existing ulcers. Mega-doses should not be administered without the recommendation of a physician or registered dietitian. Consider supplementation of a 100% recommended daily allowance (RDA) vitamin/mineral supplement that is automatically incorporated into the care plan. Supplementation beyond the RDA is not advised unless the resident has a known deficiency.[67] Vitamin and mineral assays are useful to confirm suspected deficiencies. This goes for vitamin C and zinc as well. Unless the individual has a known deficit, supplementation has not been shown to be of any benefit.

7.8 Prevention and Reimbursement

The centers for medicare and medicaid services (CMS) issued a new regulation beginning October 2008. Medicare and Medicaid will no longer provide additional reimbursement to hospitals for pressure ulcers that occurred during the patient's stay.[68] CMS believes pressure ulcers are preventable. Average extra cost for one pressure ulcer, for one patient in acute care is $40,000.[68] The challenge will be to put the law into practice without destroying our healthcare system. Success will be achieved if facilities align policies, procedures, and personnel to prevent these nosocomial events or hospital acquired conditions (HAC) from occurring and offer quality patient care. It is recommended that hospitals ramp up education and programs to prepare for these changes. This will include the development of key relationships to provide cost-effective products and programs to streamline care and save money. A similar prospective payment system has been in place within long-term care (LTC) since 2004.

7.9 Prevention, Full-Circle

Wound prevention can be equated to the care and maintenance of inanimate objects or things such as automobiles or our homes; similar to getting a "tune up" on our automobile or replacing the shingles on a house. The human body, however, is a living system, ultimately capable of healing itself and maintaining the skin barrier function with the proper prevention measures. Although a complex process, most wounds can be prevented with the right protocols, products, personnel, education, and policies and procedures. As the old adage states, "an ounce of prevention is worth a pound of cure." Not only does wound prevention save facilities and payers time, money and possible litigation, but ultimately the patient will be spared ache and anguish, increasing the quality of life.

References

1. Norman RA, Menendez R. Structure and function of aging skin. In: Norman RA, ed. *Diagnosis of Aging Skin Diseases*. London: Springer; 2008
2. Baranoski S, Ayello EA, eds. *Skin: An Essential Organ, Chapter 4 in Wound Care Essentials Practice Principles*. Philadelphia, PA: Lippincott Williams and Wilkins; 2004:49
3. Goldstein DR, et al Differential diagnosis: assessment of the lower extremity ulcer. Is it arterial, venous, neuropathic? *Wounds*. 1998;10:125–131
4. Rutherford RB. The vascular consultation. In: Rutherford RB, ed. *Vascular Surgery*. 4th ed. Philadelphia, PA: WB Saunders; 1995

5. Young JR. Differential diagnosis of leg ulcers. *Cariovasc Clin.* 1983;13(2):171–193

6. Beylin M. Treating venous stasis ulcers in the lower extremity. *Podiatry Today.* 2004;17(10):68–74

7. Fleck CA. Measuring ankle brachial index. *Adv Skin Wound Care.* 2007;20(12):645–649

8. Vowden K, Vowden P. Doppler and the ABPI: how good is our understanding? *J Wound Care.* 2001;10:197–202

9. Criqui MH, Browner D, Fronek A, et al Periperal arterial disease in large vessels is epidemiologically distinct from small vessel disease. *Am J Epidemiol.* 1989;129:1110–1119

10. Wound, Ostomy, and Continence Clinical Practice Ostomy Subcommittee. Ankle Brachial Index: Best Practice for Clinicians; 2005:1

11. Wound Ostomy Continence Nurses Society. Guidelines for Management of Wounds in Patients with Lower Extremity Arterial Disease. Glenview, IL; 2002

12. Criqui M. Systemic atherosclerosis risk and the mandate for intervention in atherosclerotic peripheral disease. *Am J Cardiol.* 2001;88(7B):433–447

13. Nelson EA, Cullum N, Jones J. Compression for preventing recurrence of venous ulcers. Cochrane Review, The Cochrane Library, Issue 2; 2003

14. Wound, Ostomy and Continence Nurses Society Guideline for Management of Wounds in Patients with Lower-Extremity Neuropathic Disease, WOCN Clinical Practice Guideline Series number 3. Glenview, IL; 2004

15. Vijay V, Saraswathy G, Gautham A, et al Effectiveness of different types of footwear insoles for the diabetic neuropathic foot. A follow-up study. *Diabet Care.* 2004;27(2): 474–477

16. Knowles EA, Boulton AJM. Do people with diabetes wear their prescribed footwear? *Diabet Med.* 1996;13:1064

17. Armstrong DG, Lavery LA, Kimbriel HR, et al Activity patterns of patients with diabetic foot ulcers: patients with active ulceration may not adhere to a standard pressure offloading regimen. *Diabet Care.* 2003;26:2595–2597

18. American Diabetes Association. Consensus Statement: Diabetes Care, Consensus Development Conference on Diabetic Foot Wound Care. Alexandria, VA; 2003

19. Birke JA, Rolfsen RJ. Evaluation of a self-administered sensory testing tool to identify patients at risk of diabetes-related foot problems. *Diabet Care.* 1998;21:23–25

20. Birke JA, Patout CA, Foto JG. Factors associated with ulceration and amputation in the neuropathic foot. *J Orthop Sports Phys Ther.* 2000;30(2):91–97

21. Dillingham T, Pezzin L, Mackenzie E. Limb amputation and limb deficiency. *South Med J.* 2002;95:875–883

22. Schainfield R. Management of peripheral arterial disease and intermittent claudication. *J Am Board Fam Pract.* 2001;14: 443–445

23. Federman DG, Trent J, Frelich C, Deinovic J, Kirsner R. Epidemiology of peripheral vascular disease: a predictor of systemic vascular disease. *Ostomy Wound Manage.* 1998;44:58–66

24. Taylor LM, Porter JM. Natural history and nonoperative treatment of chronic lower extremity ischemia. In: Moore WS, ed. *Vascular Surgery: A Comprehensive Review.* Philadelphia, PA: W.B. Saunders; 1993

25. Fleck CA. How to avoid perineal skin care problems. *Extended Care Product News.* 2004;96(6):1, 13–16

26. Hill MJ. *Dermatology Nursing Essentials: A Core Curriculum.* 2nd ed. Pittman, New Jersey: Anthony J. Jannetti Publication Management; 2003

27. Sibbald RG, Campbell K, Coutts P, Queen D. Intact skin – an integrity not to be lost. *Ost Wound Manag.* 2003;49(6):27–41

28. Nix DH. Prevention and treatment of perineal skin breakdown. In: Milne CT, Corbett LQ, Duboc D, eds. *Wound Ostomy and Continence Nursing Secrets.* Philadelphia, PA: Hanley and Belfus; 2003:373–377

29. Storer-Brown D. Perineal dermatitis: can we measure it? *Ost Wound Manag.* 1993;39(7):8–30,32

30. Nix DH. Validity and reliability of the perineal assessment tool (PAT). *Ostomy Wound Manag.* 2002;48(2):43–49

31. Wound, Ostomy and Continence Nurses Society. Guidelines for Prevention and Management of Pressure Ulcers. WOCN Clinical Practice Guidelines Series. Glenview, IL. WOCN Society; 2003:14

32. Gray M, et al Incontinence-associated dermatitis: a consensus. *J WOCN.* 2007;314(1):45–54

33. Calhoun JH, et al Diabetic foot ulcers and infections: current concepts. *Adv Skin Wound Care.* 2002;15(2):31–42

34. Bryant RA, ed. *Acute and Chronic Wounds: Nursing Management.* 2nd ed. St. Louis, MO: Mosby-Yearbook; 2000

35. Ananthapadmanabhan KP, Moore DJ, Subramanyan K, Misra M, Meyer F. Cleansing without compromise: the impact of cleansers on the skin barrier and the technology of mild cleansing. *Dermatol Ther.* 2004;17(suppl 1):16–25

36. Lutz J. Cleansing lotions vs bar soap for skin care use. Presented at the Wound Ostomy and Continence Nurses Society National Conference; 1998

37. Norman RA. Causes and management of xerosis and pruritis in the elderly. *Ann Long Term Care.* 2001;9(12):35–40

38. Fleck CA, McCord D. The dawn of advanced skin care. *Extended Care Product News.* 2004;95(5):32, 34–39

39. Fantl JA, Newman DK, Colling J, et al Managing Acute and Chronic Urinary Incontinence, Clinical Practice Guideline. Quick Reference Guide for Clinicians, No. 2, 1996 Update. Rockville, MD: U.S. Department of Health and Human Services, Public Health Service. Agency for Health Care Policy and Research. AHCPR Pub. No. 96–0686. March 1996

40. Groom M, Shannon RJ, Chakravarthy D, Fleck CA., An evaluation of cost and effects of a nutrient-based skin care program for prevention of skin tears in an extended convalescence center; accepted for publishing, *Journal of Wound, Ostomy and Continence Nursing* in press, 2010

41. Shannon RJ, Coombs M, Chakravarthy D. Reducing Hospital-Acquired Pressure Ulcers with a Siliconebased Dermal Nourishing Emollient-Associated Skincare Regimen, *Advances in Skin and Wound Care.* 2009;22(10):461–467

42. Revis DR. Decubitus Ulcers, October 2005, eMedicine at http://www.emedicine.com

43. Cuddigan J, et al, eds. *Pressure Ulcers in America: Prevalence, Incidence and Implications for the Future.* Reston, VA: National Pressure Ulcer Advisory Panel (NPUAP); 2001

44. Beckrich K, Aronovitch S. Hospital acquired pressure ulcers: a comparison of costs in medical vs. surgical patients. *Nurs Econ.* 1999;17(5):263–271

45. Young ZF, Evans A, Davis J. Nosocomial pressure ulcer prevention: a successful project. *J Nurs Adm.* 2003;33:380–383

46. Allman RM. Pressure ulcers among the elderly. *N Engl J Med.* 1989;320(13):850–853

47. National Pressure Ulcer Advisory Panel. Available at:http://www.npuap.org

48. Abrussezze RS. Early assessment and prevention of pressure ulcers. In: Lee BY, ed. *Chronic Ulcers of the Skin.* New York: McGraw-Hill; 1985:1–9

49. Kosiak M. Etiology and pathology of ischemic ulcers. *Arch Phys Med Rehabil.* 1959;40(2):62

50. Reswick J, Rogers J. *Experiences at Rancho Los Amigos Hospital with Devices and Techniques to Prevent Pressure Sores. Bedsore Biomechanics.* London: University Park; 1976

51. Walsh JS, Plonczynski DJ. Evaluation of a protocol for prevention of facility-acquired heel pressure ulcers. *JWOCN.* 2007;34(2):179

52. Coats-Bennet U. Use of support surfaces in the ICU. *Crit Care Nurs Q.* 2002;25:22–32

53. Panel for the Prediction and Prevention of Pressure Ulcers in Adults: Pressure Ulcers in Adults: Prediction and Prevention. Clinical Practice Guidelines, No. 3 AHCPR Publication No. 92–0047. Rockville, MD, Agency for Health Care Policy and Research, Public Health Service, U.S. Department of Health and Human Services, May 1992

54. Fleck C. Reducing the pressure: methods for effective wound care management. *Contin Care.* 2002;3(1):37–42

55. Kosiak M. Etiology of decubitus ulcers. *Arch Phys Med Rehabil.* 1961;42(1):19–28

56. Reddy M, Gill SS, Rochon PA. Preventing pressure ulcers: a systematic review. *JAMA.* 2006;296(8):974–984

57. Ratliff C, Bryant D. (2003) Guideline for Prevention and Management of Pressure Ulcers. WOCN Clinical Practice Guideline Series, No. 2 Wound, Ostomy and Continence Nurses Society. Available at: http://www.wocn.org

58. Duimel-Peeters I, et al The Effects of Massage to Prevent Pressure Ulcers. A Review of the Literature. *Ostomy Wound Manag.* 2005;51(4):70–80

59. Holmes A, Edelstein T. Envisioning a world without pressure ulcers. *ECPN.* 2007;122:24–29

60. Fleck CA, Sprigle S. Support surfaces: tissue integrity, terms, principles and choice (Chapter 62). In: Krasner D, Rodeheaver G, Sibbald G, eds. *Chronic Wound Care: A Clinical Sourcebook for Healthcare Professionals.* Malvern, VA, USA. 4th ed. Health Management Publications; 2007

61. Clark M. Repositioning to prevent pressure sores – what is the evidence? *Nurs Stand.* 1998;13(3):58–60, 62, 64

62. Breslow R. Nutritional status and dietary intake of patients with pressure ulcers: review of research literature 1943–1989. *Decubitus.* 1991;4:16–21

63. Pinchofsky-Devin G, Kaminski M. The correlation of pressure sores and nutritional status. *J Am Geriatr Soc.* 1986;37:173–183

64. Allman RM, Goode PS, Patrick MM, Burst N, Bartolucci AA. Pressure ulcer risk factors among hospitalized patient with activity limitation. *JAMA.* 1995;273:865–870

65. Morley J, Silver A. Nutritional issues in nursing home care. *Ann Intern Med.* 1995;123:850–859

66. Flanigan KH. Nutritional aspects of wound healing. *Adv Wound Care.* 1997;10(2):48–52

67. Thomas DR. Nutritional factors affecting wound healing. *Ostomy Wound Manag.* 1996;42(5):40–48

68. CMS Inpatient PPS Final Rule for FY 2008 available at: http://www.cms.hhs.gov.AcuteInpatientPPS/downloads/CMS-1533-FC.pdf

Helpful Websites

Association for the Advancement of Wound Care (AAWC) –www.aawconline.org

American Academy of Wound Management (AAWM) – www.aawm.org

Advancing the Practice – www.advancingthepractice.org Wound, Ostomy and Continence Nurses Association (WOCN) –www.wocn.org

Prevention of Surgical Complications

8

Michael R. Hinckley

8.1 Introduction

One of the defining characteristics of dermatology is wide array of procedures that are performed on the skin. Whether for diagnostic or treatment purposes, dermatologic procedures are an important constituent contributing to the personality of this specialty. Dermatologic surgery is one of the most important of these procedures and although not common, adverse events can result, which are troublesome both for the patient and the physician. An appropriate knowledge of how to prevent such undesirable occurrences is mandatory for any physician wishing to engage in dermatologic surgery. It is hoped that this chapter will contribute to this important body of knowledge.

8.2 Bleeding

Bleeding is an unavoidable part of any surgical procedure but a typical dermatologic surgery should involve minimal bleeding. Several steps can be taken preoperatively, perioperatively, and postoperatively to decrease the potential of bleeding.

The preoperative history should review all medications and the physician should verbally inquire about any history of abnormal bleeding or use of anticoagulant or antiplatelet medication. While some patients might be familiar with the blood thinning effects of medicines such as warfarin, heparin, aspirin, and clopidogrel, they may not realize that numerous other substances can cause thinning of the blood. Like aspirin, nonsteroidal antiinflammatory drugs (NSAIDS) act as platelet inhibitors, although in contrast to aspirin, their antiplatelet effect is reversible.[1] Other products with antiplatelet effect include alcohol, fish oil (Omega three polyunsaturated fatty acids), ginseng, gingko biloba, garlic, ginger, feverfew, vitamin E, and green tea.[1-3] As patients may not know of these products' potential to thin blood, it is prudent to specifically ask about the use of these substances. Finding purpura on physical examination can also indicate a clotting problem or use of a blood thinner.

Some patients can safely discontinue the use of some blood thinners before cutaneous surgery, and if so, they should be told how far in advance to stop the medicine. The antiplatelet effect of some common blood thinners is shown in Table 8.1.[4,5] Cutaneous surgery on a patient taking common blood thinners is considered safe and most reports have shown no increase of surgical complications.[6,7] Physicians should be aware that patients taking more than one blood thinner may be at increased risk of bleeding compared to those who took only one or no blood thinning agents.[8] In any patient with a medical necessity for warfarin, the medication should be continued through surgery.[7] Patients on aspirin that is medically necessary should also continue the medication unless the surgery will be involving "deep tissue resection or dissection."[7] If surgery is performed on a patient taking warfarin, some surgeons request an international normalized ratio (INR) between two and three unless the prescribing physician specifies otherwise.[9] One study reported safety of surgical procedures with INR of less than 3.5 and recommended preoperative testing of INR preferably within 24 h of surgery.[10]

M.R. Hinckley
Department of Dermatology,
Wake Forest University Baptist Medical Center,
Winston-Salem, NC, USA
e-mail: mhinckley@wfubmc.edu

R.A. Norman (ed.), *Common Treatments in Preventive Dermatology*,
DOI 10.1007/978-0-85729-853-9_8, © Springer-Verlag London Limited 2012

Table 8.1 Duration of blood thinning effect of various agents (days)

Aspirin	8–10
Warfarin	2–5
Clopidogrel	5

In the preoperative history, it should also be ascertained if the patient has any inherited bleeding disorders. In such patients, a hematology consultation is warranted to ensure that appropriate measures are taken to prevent excessive bleeding.[11,12]

Perioperatively, the use of the vasoconstrictor epinephrine in the local anesthetic will help decrease bleeding.[13] Moreover, absorption of the anesthetic is reduced and the risk of toxicity is lessened.[13] Methods of stopping bleeding during surgery include the use of electrosurgery, electrocautery, pressure, and tying off vessels. Hydrophilic polymers with potassium salt and microporous polysaccharide hemispheres are products that can help with hemostasis.[14] Hydrophilic polymers with potassium salt should only be used on wounds where second-intention healing will be allowed.[14]

Postoperatively covering the excision site with a pressure dressing can theoretically decrease bleeding. When bleeding does occur after surgery, a hematoma may form. Evacuation of early hematomas is advised and even if not treated early, it is still probably best to evacuate hematomas that are expanding or large and have become fibrous.[1] Observation is acceptable for a hematoma that is stable and small.[1] If control of bleeding has been difficult during performance of a large multilayered closure or flap, hematoma formation may be prevented by drain placement.[1] If an intraoral hematoma forms after surgery on the cheek, it is best to avoid intervention through the mucosa because of the risk of forming a fistula to the cheek wound on the outside.[15] Furthermore, involvement of an oral and maxillofacial surgeon is advisable.[15]

8.2.1 Key Points

- Be aware of blood thinners patients are using.
- Blood thinners used for primary prevention can be stopped.
- Do not discontinue medically necessary blood thinners.
- Evacuate early or expanding hematomas.

8.3 Infection

Dermatologic surgeons have been fortunate to enjoy a low incidence of postoperative infection. Different rates have been reported, but one recent publication found an overall infection incidence of 0.7%.[16] Patient risk factors that may affect the rate of infection are shown in Table 8.2.[17,18] While diabetes and smoking has been thought to increase infection risk, one study found no increased risk of infection in diabetics or smokers.[16] Many patient risk factors are chronic and are difficult to alter immediately prior to surgery, but those with potential risk factors that can be controlled should be. Patients with diabetes can work to achieve optimal blood glucose control and those who use tobacco or alcohol can be encouraged to decrease the amount used. Increased rate of infection can also be seen in skin grafts, ear or lip wedge resections, and in surgery performed in the groin and below the knee.[16] Other factors that might affect rate of infection include

Table 8.2 Some risk factors for infection

Male gender
Advancing age
Immunosuppression
Malnutrition
Diabetes mellitus
Obesity
Peripheral vascular disease
Alcohol use
Tobacco use
Bacterial colonization
Chronic renal insufficiency
Transfusion of blood products during surgery
Concurrent remote infection
Corticosteroid use
Skin grafts
Ear or lip wedge resections
Surgery in the groin and below the knee
Longer surgery duration
Reconstructive procedures
Surgery on the nose, ear, and facial region

longer surgery duration, reconstructive procedures, and surgery on the nose, ear, and facial region.[18] Use of prophylactic antibiotics should be considered in the proper scenarios.

Although it might be assumed that the use of sterile gloves during surgery would decrease potential for infection, not all data support this. One report has demonstrated that the use of nonsterile gloves during Mohs micrographic surgery resulted in no increased infection rates except in patients who underwent fenestration of cartilage with secondary healing and removal of melanomas.[19] Another study showed almost no difference in infection rates in simple excisions with or without sterile glove use (1.7% without sterile gloves, 1.6% with sterile gloves).[18] However, this same report found incidence of infection to be 14.7% when sterile gloves were not used in excisions with a reconstructive procedure and 3.4% with the use of sterile gloves.[18]

An advisory statement published in 2008 by physicians at the Mayo Clinic provides a number of scenarios where prophylactic antibiotics are appropriate.

- High risk of surgical site infection: lower extremity, especially leg; groin; wedge excisions of the lip or ear; skin flaps on the nose; skin grafts; extensive inflammatory skin disease.
- Prevention of infective endocarditis: Prosthetic cardiac valve, previous infective endocarditis; cardiac transplantation recipients who develop cardiac valvulopathy; congenital heart disease (CHD) (unrepaired cyanotic CHD, including palliative shunts and conduits, during the first 6 months after complete repair of congenital heart defects with prosthetic material or device placed by surgery or catheter intervention); repaired congenital heart disease with residual defects at the site or adjacent to the site of a prosthetic patch or prosthetic device (which inhibit endothelialization).
- Prevention of hematologic total joint infection: The first 2 years following joint replacement; previous prosthetic joint infections, immunocompromised/immunosuppressed patients (inflammatory arthropathies such as rheumatoid arthritis, systemic lupus erythematosus, drug- or radiation-induced immunosuppression); insulin-dependent type I diabetes; HIV infection; malignancy; malnourishment; hemophilia.[20]

The American Heart Association guidelines published in 2007 for infective endocarditis (IE) prophylaxis state that "Antibiotic prophylaxis is reasonable for procedures on respiratory tract or infected skin, skin structures, or musculoskeletal tissue only for patients with underlying cardiac conditions associated with the highest risk of adverse outcome from IE."[21] That report lists the following conditions:

- Prosthetic cardiac valve or prosthetic material used for cardiac valve repair
- Previous IE
- CHD
  - Unrepaired cyanotic CHD, including palliative shunts and conduits.
  - Completely repaired congenital heart defect with prosthetic material or device, whether placed by surgery or by catheter intervention, during the first 6 months after the procedure.
  - Repaired CHD with residual defects at the site or adjacent to the site of a prosthetic patch or prosthetic device (which inhibit endothelialization).
- Cardiac transplantation recipients who develop cardiac valvulopathy[21]

Another report listed the following noncardiac conditions as high risk: orthopedic prosthesis, central nervous system (CNS) shunts, and shunt or fistula with nearby or inflamed tissue.[17] This same report noted that antibiotic prophylaxis may be appropriate in situations such as closures with high tension, procedures performed on the hand, infected or inflamed skin of a surgical site, when a flap or graft is done on the ear and nose, and when several procedures are done at once.[17] If infection would lead to serious consequences such as in immunosuppressed patients, prophylactic antibiotics for surgery performed in the axillae and mucosal surfaces are given.[17] The American Academy of Orthopedic Surgeons website recommends prophylactic antibiotics for those who have had a joint replacement in particular scenarios if a patient is undergoing certain dental and urologic procedures.[22,23] If a patient with a prosthesis is to undergo skin surgery, the dermatologic surgeon might consider the use of preoperative antibiotics if the prosthesis was placed within the previous 2 years. However, the orthopedic surgeon who placed the prosthesis can be contacted if there is any question.

Prophylaxis should be timed appropriately to allow for adequate accumulation of the antimicrobial in the coagulum.[17] While therapy should be tailored with gram-positive organisms in mind, surgery done in moist areas, below the knees, or on diabetics might also have a high density of gram-negative organisms.[24]

When it is determined that antibiotic prophylaxis is appropriate, different regimens can be employed depending on the site. For nonoral skin, 2 g of oral cephalexin or dicloxacillin is given 0.5–1 h prior to surgery.[17] Alternatives for penicillin-allergic patients are 600 mg of oral clindamycin or 500 mg of oral azithromycin given 0.5–1 h prior to surgery.[17] For nasal and oral mucosa 2 g of oral amoxicillin or if penicillin-allergic 600 mg of oral clindamycin, 500 mg of oral azithromycin, or if nontype one reaction 2 g of oral cephalexin can be given ½–1 h prior to surgery.[17] Unless surgery lasts longer than 6 h, the preoperative dose could be sufficient for endocarditis and prosthesis prophylaxis.[17] In a patient believed to be at high risk for infection of a wound, up to 10 days of antibiotics can be given postoperatively in addition to the preoperative dose, twice a day for cephalosporins rather than four times a day.[17]

Preoperative preparation of the surgical site is a step the surgical staff can take in an effort to decrease postoperative wound infection. Chlorhexidine gluconate and povidone-iodine are antiseptics commonly employed for skin surgery. While povidone-iodine has been used as an antimicrobial for many years, it has a number of disadvantages. It might be inactivated by blood[25] and it can be toxic to human fibroblasts and thus slow the rate of wound healing.[26] Furthermore, as compared to chlorhexidine, it is more likely to cause an allergic reaction,[27] it is less effective at clearing of microbes,[28] and it has less sustained activity than chlorhexidine.[29] Chlorhexidine gluconate can also be problematic as keratopathy has been reported[30] and ototoxicity has been found with its use in animal studies.[31,32] Thus, this is probably an unwise choice for cleansing in the auricular region or to prepare the skin around the eyes. Alcohol has a rapid onset of action but duration of action is limited.[29] An optimal combination is chlorhexidine gluconate and alcohol, thus providing the potential for rapid onset and prolonged duration of action.[29] Surrounding the surgical site with sterile draping, either disposable or washable, might also help keep the area clean and prevent infection.

Postoperatively, an antibiotic ointment can be placed with an overlying dressing. Ointments include bacitracin, mupirocin, neomycin, erythromycin, polymyxin, and combinations of the different topicals.[33]

Mupirocin is effective against gram-positive and some gram-negative organisms and is less likely to cause contact dermatitis than some other topical antibiotics.[33] Neomycin is bactericidal against most gram-negatives bacteria and against staphylococci but not against streptococci.[33] Neomycin-induced allergic contact dermatitis has been reported to occur in 1–6% of people.[33] Bacitracin is effective against various gram-positive and gram-negative microbes[33] but along with neomycin can cause contact dermatitis.[34] Polymyxin is most effective at killing some gram-negative bacteria, and when used in combination with other topical antibiotics, the preparation has increased spectrum of activity.[33] Erythromycin 2% ointment has bactericidal activity against gram-positive bacteria with little risk of sensitization.[35] Silver sulfadiazine is bactericidal against gram-negative and gram-positive bacteria.[33] Retapamulin is a topical antibiotic for the treatment of impetigo with activity against Streptococcus pyogenes and Staphylococcus aureus.[36]

Petrolatum can be used as an alternative to antibiotic ointment following surgery. One study was unable to find a statistically significant difference in the rate of postoperative infections in patients who had used white petrolatum vs. bacitracin (2% vs. 0.9%).[37] Moreover, there was no difference in healing that was clinically significant noted at day 1, 7, or 28.[37] No contact dermatitis was seen in the white petrolatum group.[37] In addition, anaphylaxis to bacitracin has been reported.[38] Another study found no statistically significant difference between petrolatum and gentamycin ointment in prevention of postoperative suppurative auricular chondritis.[39] Furthermore, inflammatory chondritis was much more likely in patients who used gentamycin ointment compared to petrolatum.[39]

In light of the potential for side effects and resistance, as well as the lack of strict guidelines for antibiotic use in skin surgery, the need for oral and topical antibiotics should be determined on a case-by-case basis.

8.3.1 Key Points

- Infection in dermatologic surgery is low.
- Petrolatum can be safely used on postoperative sites instead of antibiotic ointment.
- Use antibiotic prophylaxis when appropriate.

8.4 Allergic Reactions

Every preoperative medical history should elicit information about drug allergies. Adverse drug reactions can range from mild annoyances to fatalities. A study looking at adverse drug events estimated that over 700,000 people in the United States are treated annually in emergency departments for such events.[40] While few medications are used in conjunction with dermatologic surgery, the surgeon should be aware of those that are most likely to be problematic (Table 8.3). Semisynthetic penicillinase-resistant penicillins and first-generation cephalosporins are the most common antibiotics used for prophylaxis in skin surgery.[41] Although 0.7–10% claim such an allergy, of these individuals around 10–30% show a positive IgE-mediated reaction on skin testing.[42] Although cross-reactivity between cephalosporins and penicillin can occur, it is probably less than once thought.[43] Historically, 10% cross-reactivity has been reported, but this number may have resulted from penicillin compounds that were contaminated with cephalosporins.[43] Approximately 1–3% of patients can experience an allergic or immune-mediated reaction to cephalosporins.[43] If a patient does have a penicillin or cephalosporin allergy and an antibiotic is warranted, clindamycin can be used as an alternative.[17]

Antiseptics can also cause an allergic reaction in dermatologic surgery. Povidone-iodine-containing antiseptics are the most common antiseptics to cause allergic contact dermatitis.[27] Anaphylaxis due to the povidone component of povidone-iodine has been reported.[44]

Local anesthetics used in cutaneous surgery typically belong to the amide class of anesthetics. Allergy to local anesthetics is rare, particularly among the amide class.[45-47] Anesthetics from the ester class are more likely to cause a reaction than those from the amide class and this is due to p-aminobenzoic acid, an

Table 8.3 Potential allergens in a surgical setting

Antibiotics (oral and topical)
Antiseptics
Anesthetic
Latex
Nickel (surgical instruments)
Suture
Colophony (adhesive tape)

ester metabolite.[27] Patients can experience side effects from epinephrine, which is sometimes mixed with anesthetic and such adverse affects are more likely in patients with hyperthyroidism, significant cardiac disease, who are very anxious or who are taking a nonselective beta-blocker.[48] Such reactions include palpitations, tachycardia, tremor, headache, diaphoresis, chest pain, nervousness, light-headedness, and increased blood pressure.[48] If a patient is worried about side effects of epinephrine or has a condition that could result in increased sensitivity to epinephrine, the surgeon should discuss the adverse effects of the epinephrine with the patient and decide if anesthetic without epinephrine would be preferable. If epinephrine is not used, the surgeon and the patient should understand that bleeding will likely be greater and the duration of the anesthetic effect will probably be shorter.

Perioperative allergic reactions can result from rubber products (such as latex), acrylates (found in electrosurgical plates), formaldehyde (formaldehyde gas emanating from an open biopsy specimen container), nickel (found in surgical instruments), and suture (prolene allergy is rare but has been reported).[27]

Postoperative contact dermatitis can result from adhesives and topical antibiotics.[27] Both neomycin and bacitracin were listed among the top ten allergens in a Mayo Clinic report investigating allergens over a 5-year period.[34] These same two topicals were among the top ten relevant allergens in an investigation of causes of allergic contact dermatitis in patients with hand dermatitis.[49] Use of these medications may give a postsurgical wound the appearance of infection when the true issue is contact allergy. Bacitracin-induced anaphylaxis has been reported.[38] Petrolatum can be considered for use on surgical sites in place of topical antibiotics.

Adhesive tape can contain colophony, a cause of contact dermatitis.[27] Band-aid Liquid Bandage and Dermabond contain 2-octyl cyanoacrylate and colorant,[27] and benzalkonium chloride and methylparaben are also found in Liquid Bandage[27]; these four sensitizers can result in allergy.[27]

Physicians should be aware of patient allergies and be able to recognize allergic reactions, which could result in misdiagnosis of the real problem. For example, if a patient returns to clinic after surgery for suture removal and the surgical area appears inflamed, the cause may be a reaction to the topical antibiotic or tape used postoperatively and not due to infection.

Diagnosing an allergic response as infection could lead to improper use of antibiotics.

8.4.1 Key Points

- Local anesthetics rarely cause true allergic reactions.
- Potential allergens use in cutaneous surgery include latex, povidone-iodine, adhesive, suture, antibiotics.
- Inflammation at a surgical site may be secondary to a topical antibiotic.

8.5 Postoperative Scars, Pain, and Pruritus

Scarring is an inevitable result of surgery and should be expected in all cases. While several steps can be taken to minimize the size and appearance of surgical scars, during the explanation of the surgical procedure and in the informed consent, it should be made clear to the patient that a scar will result. Location can affect how a scar forms[50] and the physician may want to inform the patient of this. In the preoperative assessment, a patient should be asked about history of hypertrophic scarring or keloid formation. Physical examination is also helpful as a hypertrophic scar, or keloid might be noted by the physician that was not mentioned by the patient.

A variety of patient-related factors can affect scar outcome. Sun exposure can worsen the appearance of scars.[51] Diabetes is a risk factor for infection[17] and infection can affect wound healing and result in a poor scar.[1] One study found that the most significant patient risk factors contributing to wound complications following skin biopsy appeared to be corticosteroid use and cigarette smoking.[52] Nicotine acts as a vasoconstrictor resulting in ischemia.[52] Avoidance of vigorous activities helps with split thickness skin graft survival,[53] and thus it might be assumed that refraining from such activity after other types of surgical repair will aid in healing. It seems that poor nutrition can affect healing as certain nutrients appear to be important for proper healing.[54,55] Corticosteroid use can affect healing[56,57], presumably due to the affect on the inflammatory response.[56] Chronic alcohol intake may negatively affect wound healing by decreasing activity and proliferation of T cells.[58] Stress can possibly result in poorer wound healing by affecting cytokine production.[59,60] It could be concluded that any factor that can affect wound healing will, as a result, have the potential to affect the scar formation.

Several physician-influenced factors can affect scar outcome. Perioperative handling of tissue can affect scarring.[61] High tension of a wound can result in scar spread[1] and choice of repair can influence tension. Suture track scars are more likely to develop the longer they are left in place.[1] If wound edges are not everted, the scar that forms may be more noticeable.[62] Wound separation can result from a hematoma[1], which could lead to a poor scar; thus, inadequately controlling bleeding intraoperatively could ultimately affect the scar. Putting suture lines on the boundary of a cosmetic subunit can help with scar formation[63], and how the excision is placed in relation to relaxed skin tension lines can affect cosmesis.[63]

Management options for keloids and hypertrophic scars include interferon or corticosteroid injections, occlusive dressings, radiotherapy, compression therapy, cryotherapy, laser, surgical excision, dermabrasion, surgical revision, fillers, peels, cryosurgery, cosmetics, punch excisions and grafts, pressure bandages, and massage.[50,64] Approximately 3 weeks after surgery, a patient can massage the surgical site in an effort to achieve improved scar appearance. Topical preparations to help scars are available but one study has demonstrated no advantage of an onion extract-based gel over a petrolatum-based ointment.[65] Use of a silicone gel cushion and silicone sheeting for hypertrophic scars and keloids has resulted in decreased volume and symptoms of scars.[64] Silicone elastomer sheeting appears to be useful in the prevention and treatment of keloid scars and hypertrophic scars.[66] It may be that hydration rather than silicone is what is helping.[67] Patients should be warned that scar maturation can take up to 1 year and improvement can be seen up until that time. Proper education of patients and skillful surgeons can do much to achieve acceptable scars for patients.

Pain, pruritus, and numbness of surgical sites are benign but relatively common symptoms reported by patients. Some topical treatments might improve symptoms. Retinoic acid applied daily to hypertrophic and keloid scars has been reported to decrease pruritus and tenderness, and tocoretinate ointment has resulted in decreased pruritus in mature hypertrophic scars.[68] Silicone-containing products used for hypertrophic scars and keloids have resulted in decreased tenderness and pruritus.[64] Topical lidocaine could also be tried for symptomatic relief of scars.

Postoperative pain in dermatologic surgery will rarely be a serious problem. After simple excisions and repairs, acetaminophen should be adequate to control pain. Patients should be warned that other over-the-counter painkillers such as aspirin, ibuprofen, naproxen, or other NSAIDS can cause bleeding. In larger excisions or more advanced repairs, patients might need a prescription for stronger analgesics. If a prescription is given for a compound containing acetaminophen, the patient should be warned that use of the prescription medication in addition to acetaminophen could result in toxicity.

8.5.1 Key Points

- Tension, bleeding, infection, and vigorous activity can result in an undesirable scar.
- Placing an incision within relaxed skin tension lines can help hide a scar.
- Occlusive dressings, massage, corticosteroid injection can improve scar appearance.
- Protect scars from the sun.

8.6 Standing Cones

Standing cones ("dog ears") are more likely to result when length-to-width ratio of a fusiform excision is less than 3–4:1, when opposing sides of a wound are of unequal length, or if the angles at the wound apices are too big.[69] Too much tension can cause depression of the center of the wound and the skin at the ends to be elevated, thus giving the look of dog ears.[69] Inadequate undermining can accentuate dog ears and if during a fusiform excision the scalpel angle is not at 90° while approaching the apices, dog ears can result.[69] Standing cones can sometimes resolve over time.[70]

8.6.1 Key Points

- Can result from too much tension, inadequate undermining, when length-to-width ratio is less than 3:1.
- Standing cones can sometimes resolve over time.

8.7 Anesthetic Toxicity

Although local anesthesia is safer than general anesthesia,[71] toxicity can result, and the CNS and cardiovascular system are the two main organ systems where adverse reactions occur[72] (Table 8.4). CNS side effects include circumoral numbness, light-headedness, double vision, a metallic taste, tremors, slurred speech, respiratory arrest, and seizure.[72] Cardiovascular effects include hypotension, dysrhythmias, palpitations, shortness of breath, diaphoresis, and chest pain.[73] Epinephrine can cause several side effects (Table 8.5) and should be used cautiously in patients on a beta-blocker and with heart disease.[13] Conversing with the patient during surgery may allow the physician to identify toxicity by noticing problems such as a change in mental status or dysarthria.[74]

Epinephrine is helpful in the setting of local anesthetic as its use results in less absorption of the anesthetic, the need for a smaller amount of the anesthetic, and decreased risk of toxicity.[13] Absorption of anesthetic also depends on the vascularity of the area being injected.[75] Aspirating

Table 8.4 Symptoms of anesthetic toxicity

Central nervous system	Cardiovascular
Circumoral numbness	Hypotension
Light-headedness	Dysrhythmias
Double vision	Palpitations
Metallic taste	Shortness of breath
Tremors	Diaphoresis
Slurred speech	Chest pain
Respiratory arrest	
Seizure	

Table 8.5 Potential side effects of epinephrine

Palpitations
Tachycardia
Tremor
Headache
Diaphoresis
Chest pain
Nervousness
Light-headedness
Increased blood pressure

during injection can reduce the chance of injecting a large amount of the anesthetic intravascularly.[74] Recommended maximum doses of anesthetic are: 4–5 mg/kg alone and 7 mg/kg with epinephrine for lidocaine, and 175 mg alone and 225 mg with epinephrine for bupivacaine.[73] Bupivacaine has the advantage of a longer duration of action but also can be particularly cardiotoxic.[73] Lidocaine is metabolized by the liver, and thus hepatic dysfunction can lead to increased risk of toxicity.[74] Local anesthetics are predominantly excreted in urine,[72] but renal failure does not lead to decreased clearance because of inactivation of amides in the liver and hydrolysis of esters in the plasma.[75]

If toxicity does occur, supportive care and crash cart materials should be available.

8.7.1 Key Points

- Talking to a patient during surgery can help the physician become aware of anesthetic toxicity such as slurred speech.
- Epinephrine can decrease absorption of the anesthetic, thus decreasing the risk of toxicity.
- Hepatic failure can increase toxicity due to decrease metabolization of the anesthetic.

8.8 Nerve Damage

Nerve damage can be one of the most devastating results of cutaneous surgery. Sensory deficits will be suffered in many cases but sensory nerves frequently regenerate though it may be some months.[76] Injury to sensory nerves resulting in permanent paresthesia or injury to motor nerves resulting in functional impairment can be more problematic. Unfortunately, excision of large or infiltrative tumors may make damage of certain nerves unavoidable. When a tumor is not large or infiltrative but located in the vicinity of an important nerve, the solution to preventing nerve damage is to have an appropriate knowledge of anatomy, particularly in the facial and neck regions.

The superficial muscularoaponeurotic system (SMAS) is a useful landmark in the face as sensory nerves ordinarily course through the superficial portion of the SMAS while motor nerves course through the deeper part of the SMAS.[63] The SMAS is typically found above the muscles but deep to the subcutaneous tissue.[63] The predominant source of sensory innervation to the face is the fifth cranial nerve or trigeminal nerve.[63] The trigeminal nerve branches into the ophthalmic, maxillary, and mandibular portions.[63] Cranial nerve seven or the facial nerve supplies muscles of facial expression with motor innervation.[63] The temporal branch provides innervation to the muscles of the upper face and transection of this branch results in lack of ability to elevate the eyebrow and in ptosis.[63] This nerve passes superficially over the middle part of the zygoma rendering it susceptible to injury.[63] The marginal mandibular nerve runs superficially near the chin and mandible, and transection leads to a droopy lip and drooling.[63] The spinal accessory nerve is susceptible to injury when surgery is being performed on the neck and can result in arm, shoulder and girdle weakness, shoulder sagging, and scapula winging.[77] Various methods for locating this nerve have been described.[77] One technique is to obliquely stroke a needle over the lateral neck, marking the hyperaesthetic points, then connect these points, which can indicate the course of the nerve.[77]

Local anesthetics work rapidly on unmyelinated sensory fibers but over time, myelinated motor fibers can also be affected resulting in temporary paralysis of facial muscle.[63] Both the surgeon and the patient should be aware of this possibility to avoid unnecessary concern.

While nerve damage can result in morbidity, proper patient education can mitigate the emotional affect if such injury does occur. If tumor size, type or location makes it possible that excision will result in nerve damage, the patient should be warned what the affect of surgery may be prior to the procedure. Through proper education of patients and vigilant attention to nerve identification and surgical technique, undesired outcomes from nerve damage can be avoided or minimized.

8.8.1 Key Points

- Damage to nerves such as the temporal branch of the facial nerve, the marginal mandibular nerve, and the spinal accessory nerve can result in important loss of function for patients.
- If a tumor is located in the vicinity of nerves that can result in impairment, the patient needs to be forewarned of this possibility.

- Local anesthetics can result in temporary paralysis of nerves.
- Transected sensory nerves can regenerate but may require months to do so.

8.9 Spitting Sutures

Spitting sutures do not pose a serious problem but can be a nuisance for patients. Superficial placement of suture may increase the possibility of spitting.[78] Monofilament absorbable suture is less reactive than vicryl and may be less likely to result in spitting.[79] Spitting sutures can be gently removed by the physician if troublesome to the patient.

8.9.1 Key Points

- Superficial placement of sutures may increase the likelihood of spitting sutures.
- Monofilament absorbable suture may be less likely than vicryl to result in spitting.

8.10 Defibrillators and Pacemakers

Electrosurgery is used as a primary method of hemostasis in dermatologic surgery. Although use of electrosurgery in most patients does not seem to result in major complications, it has been reported to cause firing of implantable cardioverter-defibrillators (ICDs) and pacemaker reprogramming.[80] Interference has been reported with electrocautery use[80] but because no electrical current is generated with this method, it should be considered a safe alternative to electrosurgery in a patient with a pacemaker or ICD. Other precautions when operating on someone with a pacemaker or ICD may include the use of short bursts, low voltage, bipolar forceps, and avoiding electrosurgery in the area of the device.[80,81] Preoperative consultation with a cardiologist should be considered if there are any concerns or questions.

8.10.1 Key Point

- In patients with pacemakers or defibrillators, electrocautery is a safe alternative to electrosurgery for hemostasis.

8.11 Trap Door (Pincushioning) Deformities

Trapdoor deformity is the bulging of tissue seen in C-, V-, or U-shaped scars and may be due to a variety of causes, including scar contracture, hypertrophy, and excessive tissue.[82] It seems that this problem may be related to undermining.[83,84] The bilobed flap is a repair design that can lead to pincushioning but the rhombic bilobed flap may decrease the incidence of pincushion-ing.[85] It has also been suggested that pincushioning secondary to the bilobed flap repair may be minimized if transposition of each flap is only 45° for a total of 90–100°.[86] This defect may also be more likely to occur with flaps in the medial or superior portion of the face.[84]

8.11.1 Key Point

- Adequate undermining may decrease the likelihood of trapdoor deformities.

8.12 Flap and Graft Necrosis

Skin flaps and grafts allow dermatologic surgeons to close large surgical defects in a way that results in optimal cosmesis. Unfortunately, flaps and grafts may necrose and compromise cosmetic outcome. However, steps can be taken to decrease the risk of necrosis. Patients smoking a pack or more a day have been found to have an increased risk of full-thickness graft or flap necrosis compared to those who never smoked or those who smoked less than a pack a day.[87] While some patients may not be willing to quit smoking prior to surgery, the surgeon should at least encourage the patient to try to decrease the amount smoked for a period both before and after surgery. Skin tension can predispose a flap to some necrosis[88] and flap design should attempt to limit the amount of tension of the repair. Delicate surgical technique has been employed to decrease the likelihood of necrosis.[89] Bolsters may be used but may not be needed for securing of full-thickness skin grafts in order to decrease the chance of necrosis.[89] Full-thickness skin grafts are more likely to necrose than split thickness grafts and necrosis is more likely in composite grafts than other graft types.[53] Recipient-site blood supply affects survival of a graft.[53]

8.12.1 Key Points

- Encourage smokers with a flap or graft to decrease smoking, at least while the defect is healing.
- Limit tension in repairs involving a flap or graft.
- Recipient site blood supply can affect the viability of a graft.

8.13 Vasovagal Reaction

A vasovagal reaction can result in patient harm if the patient falls and strikes a body part. In one study, 1% of surgical patients experienced vasovagal syncope, which occurred before, during, and after surgery.[90] Fear, emotional stress, or acute pain may be triggers but the cause is often not identified.[47] Skin may become cool and pale, bradycardia may follow tachycardia, blood pressure may drop initially, and acute brief loss of consciousness may occur.[47] If a vasovagal reaction occurs, patient should be placed in a recumbent position.[47]

8.13.1 Key Points

- Vasovagal reactions can occur in surgery patients, which can result in patient harm due to falling.
- Patients who experience a vasovagal reaction should be placed in a recumbent position.

8.14 Litigation

Perhaps every physician in the United States is affected in some way by litigation. Whether by the indirect effect of malpractice costs or the direct effect of utilizing resources to confront a lawsuit, litigation can be an influential aspect of medical practice. While preventing complications should help prevent lawsuits, other steps can be taken that might aid in avoiding litigation. Communication with patients and families, record keeping, informed consent, and availability of the attending doctor or an associate can potentially prevent lawsuits.[91] While attention to all of these details is important, a good physician-patient relationship is likely the best way to prevent litigation.[92] Such relationships between dermatologic surgeons and their patients should be an important part of every surgical practice.

8.14.1 Key Point

- Communication and a good physician–patient relationship can help avoid litigation.

8.15 Conclusion

Dermatologic surgery has proven to be a safe and effective method for treating skin disease. With a proper understanding of this field of medicine and by taking appropriate precautions, the majority of significant surgical complications can be kept to a minimum. Such practices will result in satisfying outcomes for physicians and healthier, happier patients.

References

1. Stasko T, Henghold WB. Complications in cutaneous procedures. In: Roenigk RK, Ratz JL, Roenigk HH Jr, eds. *Roenigk's Dermatologic Surgery: Current Techniques in Procedural Dermatology*. 3 rd ed. New York: Informa Healthcare; 2007
2. Mukamal KJ, Massaro JM, Ault KA, et al Alcohol consumption and platelet activation and aggregation among women and men: the Framingham offspring study alcoholism. *Alcohol Clin Exp Res*. 2005;29(10):1906–1912
3. Baldassarre D, Amato M, Eligini S, et al Effect of n-3 fatty acids on carotid atherosclerosis and haemostasis in patients with combined hyperlipoproteinemia: a double-blind pilot study in primary prevention. *Ann Med*. 2006;38(5):367–375
4. Furst DE, Ulrich RW. Nonsteroidal antiinflammatory drugs, disease-modifying antirheumatic drugs, nonopioid analgesics, and drugs used in gout. In: Katzung BG, ed. *Basic and Clinical Pharmacology*. 10th ed. New York: McGraw Hill Medical; 2007

5. Wickersham RM, Novak KK, eds. *Drug Facts and Comparisons 2008*. St. Louis, MO: Wolters Kluwer Health; 2007

6. Alcalay J, Alkalay R. Controversies in perioperative management of blood thinners in dermatologic surgery: continue or discontinue? *Dermatol Surg*. 2004;30(8):1091–1094

7. Otley CC. Continuation of medically necessary aspirin and warfarin during cutaneous surgery. *Mayo Clin Proc*. 2003; 78(11):1392–1396

8. Shimizu I, Jellinek NJ, Dufresne RG, et al Multiple antithrombotic agents increase the risk of postoperative hemorrhage in dermatologic surgery. *J Am Acad Dermatol*. 2008; 58(5):810–816

9. Kirkorian AY, Moore BL, Siskind J, Marmur ES. Perioperative management of anticoagulant therapy during cutaneous surgery: 2005 survey of Mohs surgeons. *Dermatol Surg*. 2007;33(10):1189–1197

10. Ah-Weng A, Natarajan S, Velangi S, Langtry JA. Preoperative monitoring of warfarin in cutaneous surgery. *Br J Dermatol*. 2003;149(2):386–389

11. Leonard AL, Hanke CW, Greist A. Perioperative management of von Willebrand disease in dermatologic surgery. *Dermatol Surg*. 2007;33(4):403–409

12. Peterson SR, Joseph AK. Inherited bleeding disorders in dermatologic surgery. *Dermatol Surg*. 2001;27(10):885–889

13. Koay J, Orengo I. Application of local anesthetics in dermatologic surgery. *Dermatol Surg*. 2002;28(2):143–148

14. Ho J, Hruza G. Hydrophilic polymers with potassium salt and microporous polysaccharides for use as hemostatic agents. *Dermatol Surg*. 2007;33(12):1430–1433

15. Cohen SN, Sidebottom AJ, Varma S. Intraoral hematoma: a novel complication of dermatologic surgery. *Dermatol Surg*. 2007;33(9):1139–1141

16. Maragh SL, Brown MD. Prospective evaluation of surgical site infection rate among patients with Mohs micrographic surgery without the use of prophylactic antibiotics. *J Am Acad Dermatol*. 2008;59(2):275–278

17. Maragh SL, Otley CC, Roenigk RK, Phillips PK. Antibiotic prophylaxis in dermatologic surgery: updated guidelines. *Dermatol Surg*. 2005;31(1):91-93

18. Rogues AM, Lasheras A, Amici JM, et al. Infection control practices and infectious complications in dermatological surgery. *J Hosp Infect*. 2007;65(3):258–263

19. Rhinehart MB, Murphy MM, Farley MF, et al. Sterile versus nonsterile gloves during Mohs micrographic surgery: infection rate is not affected. *Dermatol Surg*. 2006;32(6):819–826

20. Wright TI, Baddour LM, Berbari EF, et al. Antibiotic prophylaxis in dermatologic surgery: advisory statement 2008. *J Am Acad Dermatol*. 2008;59(3):464–473

21. Wilson W, Taubert KA, Gewitz M, et al. Prevention of infective endocarditis: guidelines from the American Heart Association: a guideline from the American Heart Association Rheumatic Fever, Endocarditis, and Kawasaki Disease Committee, Council on Cardiovascular Disease in the Young, and the Council on Clinical Cardiology, Council on Cardiovascular Surgery and Anesthesia, and the Quality of Care and Outcomes Research Interdisciplinary Working Group. *Circulation*. 2007;116(15):1736–1754

22. American Academy of Orthopaedic Surgeons. Dental Work After a Joint Replacement. At: http://orthoinfo.aaos.org/ topic.cfm?; topic = A002262007 Accessed 12.12.07

23. American Academy of Orthopaedic Surgeons. Your Joint Replacement: Urological Procedures and Antibiotics. At: http://orthoinfo.aaos.org/topic.cfm?topic=A00383; 2007 Accessed 12.12.07

24. Messingham MJ, Arpey CJ. Update on the use of antibiotics in cutaneous surgery. *Dermatol Surg*. 2005;31(8 Pt 2): 1068–1078

25. Ritter MA, French ML, Eitzen HE, Gioe TJ. The antimicrobial effectiveness of operative-site preparative agents: a microbiological and clinical study. *J Bone Joint Surg Am*. 1980;62:826–828

26. Balin AK, Pratt L. Dilute povidone-iodine solutions inhibit human skin fibroblast growth. *Dermatol Surg*. 2002;28(3): 210–214

27. Jacob SE, Amado A, Cohen DE. Dermatologic surgical implications of allergic contact dermatitis. *Dermatol Surg*. 2005;31(9 Pt 1):1116–1123

28. Garibaldi RA, Skolnick D, Lerer T, et al. The impact of preoperative skin disinfection on preventing intraoperative wound contamination. *Infect Control Hosp Epidemiol*. 1988;9(3):109–113

29. Spann CT, Taylor S, Weinberg J. Topical antimicrobial agents in dermatology. *Dis Mon*. 2004;50(7):407–421

30. Varley GA, Meisler DM, Benes SC, et al. Hibiclens keratopathy. A clinicopathologic case report. *Cornea*. 1990;9(4): 341–346

31. Perez R, Freeman S, Sohmer H, Sichel J Y. Vestibular and cochlear ototoxicity of topical antiseptics assessed by evoked potentials. *Laryngoscope*. 2000;110(9):1522–1527

32. Igarashi Y, Oka Y. Vestibular ototoxicity following intratympanic applications of chlorhexidine gluconate in the cat. *Arch Otorhinolaryngol*. 1988;245(4):210–217

33. Spann CT, Tutrone WD, Weinberg JM, et al. Topical antibacterial agents for wound care: a primer. *Dermatol Surg*. 2003;29(6):620-626

34. Mayo Clinic. Top Ten Contact Dermatitis Allergens Identified in Mayo Clinic Study. At: http://www.mayoclinic. org/news2006-rst/3268.html; 2007 Accessed 12.12.07

35. Bernstein SC, Roenigk RK. Surgical pearl: erythromycin ointment for topical antibiotic wound care. *J Am Acad Dermatol*. 1995;32:659–660

36. Orange A, van der Wouden J, Konig S, et al. Retapamulin ointment for the treatment of impetigo in adults and children: results of a phase III, placebo-controlled, double-blind trial. *J Am Acad Dermatol*. 2007;56(suppl 2):AB4

37. Smack DP, Harrington AC, Dunn C, et al. Infection and allergy incidence in ambulatory surgery patients using a white petrolatum vs. bacitracin ointment: a randomized controlled trial. *JAMA*. 1996;276(12):972–977

38. James WD. Use of antibiotic-containing ointment versus plain petrolatum during and after clean cutaneous surgery. *J Am Acad Dermatol*. 2006;55(5):915–916

39. Campbell RM, Perlis CS, Fisher E, Gloster HM Jr. Gentamicin ointment versus petrolatum for management of auricular wounds. *Dermatol Surg*. 2005;31(6):664–669

40. Budnitz DS, Pollock DA, Weidenbach KN, et al. National surveillance of emergency department visits for outpatient adverse drug events. *JAMA*. 2006;296:1858–1866

41. Billingsley E. The Role of Antibiotics in Cutaneous Surgery. Emedicine Oct 14, 2006. At: http://www.emedicine.com/ derm/topic821.htm; 2007 Accessed 18.12.07

42. Dodek P, Phillips P. Questionable history of immediate-type hypersensitivity to penicillin in staphylococcal endocarditis: treatment based on skin-test results versus empirical alternative treatment – a decision analysis. *Clin Infect Dis.* 1999;29(5):1251–1256

43. Pichichero ME. Cephalosporins can be prescribed safely for penicillin-allergic patients. *J Fam Pract.* 2006;55(2): 106–112

44. Adachi A, Fukunaga A, Hayashi K, et al. Anaphylaxis to polyvinylpyrrolidone after vaginal application of povidone-iodine. *Contact Derm.* 2003;48(3):133–136

45. Berkun Y, Ben-Zvi A, Levy Y, et al. Evaluation of adverse reactions to local anesthetics: experience with 236 patients. *Ann Allergy Asthma Immunol.* 2003;91(4):342–345

46. Amsler E, Flahault A, Mathelier-Fusade P, Aractingi S. Evaluation of rechallenge in patients with suspected lidocaine allergy. *Dermatology.* 2004;208:109–111

47. Fader DJ, Johnson TM. Medical issues and emergencies in the dermatology office. *J Am Acad Dermatol.* 1997;36(1): 1–16

48. The American Academy of Dermatology Joint AAD/ASDS Liaison Committee. Current issues in dermatologic office-based surgery. The American Academy of Dermatology Joint AAD/ASDS Liaison Committee. *Dermatol Surg.* 1999; 25(10):806–815

49. Warshaw EM, Ahmed RL, Belsito DV, et al. North American Contact Dermatitis Group. Contact dermatitis of the hands: cross-sectional analyses of North American Contact Dermatitis Group data, 1994–2004. *J Am Acad Dermatol.* 2007;57(2):301–314

50. American Academy of Dermatology. What is a Scar. At: http://www.aad.org/public/Publications/pamphlets/WhatisaScar.htm; 2007 Accessed 12.12.07

51. Due E, Rossen K, Sorensen LT, et al. Effect of UV irradiation on cutaneous cicatrices: a randomized, controlled trial with clinical, skin reflectance, histological, immunohistochemical and biochemical evaluations. *Acta Derm Venereol.* 2007;87(1):27–32

52. Wahie S, Lawrence CM. Wound complications following diagnostic skin biopsies in dermatology inpatients. *Arch Dermatol.* 2007;143(10):1267–1271

53. Adams DC, Ramsey ML. Grafts in dermatologic surgery: review and update on full- and split-thickness skin grafts, free cartilage grafts, and composite grafts. *Dermatol Surg.* 2005;31(8 Pt 2):1055–1067

54. Lazareth I, Hubert S, Michon-Pasturel U, Priollet P. Vitamin C deficiency and leg ulcers. A case control study. *J Mal Vasc.* 2007;32(2):96–99

55. Rojas AI, Phillips TJ. Patients with chronic leg ulcers show diminished levels of vitamins A and E, carotenes, and zinc. *Dermatol Surg.* 1999;25(8):601–604

56. Wicke C, Halliday B, Allen D, et al. Effects of steroids and retinoids on wound healing. *Arch Surg.* 2000;135:1265–1270

57. Dostal GH, Gamelli RL. The differential effect of corticosteroids on wound disruption strength in mice. *Arch Surg.* 1990;125(5):636–640

58. Gordon AJ, Olstein J, Conigliaro J. Identification and treatment of alcohol use disorders in the perioperative period. *Postgrad Med.* 2006;119(2):46–55

59. Kiecolt-Glaser JK, Loving TJ, Stowell JR, et al. Hostile marital interactions, proinflammatory cytokine production, and wound healing. *Arch Gen Psychiatry.* 2005;2(12):1377–1384

60. Glaser R, Kiecolt-Glaser JK, Marucha PT, et al. Stress-related changes in proinflammatory cytokine production in wounds. *Arch Gen Psychiatry.* 1999;56(5):450–456

61. Chen MA, Davidson TM. Scar management: prevention and treatment strategies. *Curr Opin Otolaryngol Head Neck Surg.* 2005;13(4):242–247

62. Zitelli JA. Wound healing by second intention. In: Roenigk RK, Ratz JL, Roenigk HH Jr, eds. *Roenigk's Dermatologic Surgery: Current Techniques in Procedural Dermatology.* 3 rd ed. New York: Informa Healthcare; 2007

63. Orengo I, Iyengar V. Anatomy in cutaneous surgery. Emedicine. December 15, 2006. At: http://www.emedicine.com/derm/topic820.htm; 2007 Accessed 12.12.07

64. Berman B, Flores F. Comparison of a silicone gel-filled cushion and silicon gel sheeting for the treatment of hypertrophic or keloid scars. *Dermatol Surg.* 1999;25(6):484–486

65. Chung VQ, Kelley L, Marra D, Jiang SB. Onion extract gel versus petrolatum emollient on new surgical scars: a prospective double-blinded study. *Dermatol Surg.* 2006;32(2): 193–197

66. Berman B, Perez OA, Konda S, et al. A review of the biologic effects, clinical efficacy, and safety of silicone elastomer sheeting for hypertrophic and keloid scar treatment and management. *Dermatol Surg.* 2007;33(11):1291–1302

67. Chang CC, Kuo YF, Chiu HC, et al. Hydration, not silicone, modulates the effects of keratinocytes on fibroblasts. *J Surg Res.* 1995;59:705–711

68. Zurada JM, Kriegel D, Davis IC. Topical treatments for hypertrophic scars. *J Am Acad Dermatol.* 2006;55(6):1024–1031

69. Weisberg NK, Nehal KS, Zide BM. Dog-ears: a review. *Dermatol Surg.* 2000;26(4):363–370

70. Lee KS, Kim NG, Jang P Y, et al. Statistical analysis of surgical dog-ear regression. *Dermatol Surg.* 2008;34(8): 1070–1076

71. Robinson JK. The eye and eyelid. In: Roenigk RK, Ratz JL, Roenigk HH Jr, eds. *Roenigk's Dermatologic Surgery: Current Techniques in Procedural Dermatology.* 3 rd ed. New York: Informa Healthcare; 2007

72. Revis DR, Seagle MB. Local anesthetics. Emedicine. October 26, 2005. At: http://www.emedicine.com/ent/topic20.htm; 2007 Accessed 12.12.07

73. Zamanian RT, Olsson JK, Ginther B. Toxicity, local anesthetics. Emedicine. June 20, 2005. At: http://www.emedicine.com/emerg/topic761.htm; 2007 Accessed 12.12.07

74. Peralta R, Bastings E, Guzofski S. Toxicity, Lidocaine. April 25, 2007. Emedicine. At: http://www.emedicine.com/med/topic1297.htm; 2007 Accessed 12.12.07

75. Cox B, Durieux ME, Marcus MA. Toxicity of local anaesthetics. *Best Pract Res Clin Anaesthesiol.* 2003;17(1): 111–136

76. Stasko S, Clayton AS. Surgical complications and optimizing outcomes. In: Bolognia JL, Jorizzo JL, Rapini RP, eds. *Dermatology.* New York: Mosby; 2003

77. Fisher DA. A simple method of identifying the spinal accessory nerve. *Dermatol Surg.* 2000;26(4):384–386

78. Alam M, Goldberg LH. Two-lobed advancement flap for cutaneous helical rim defects. *Dermatol Surg.* 2003;29(10): 1044–1049

79. See A, Smith HR. Partially buried horizontal mattress suture: modification of the Haneke-Marini suture. *Dermatol Surg.* 2004;30(12 Pt 1):1491–1492

80. El-Gamal HM, Dufresne RG, Saddler K. Electrosurgery, pacemakers and ICDs: a survey of precautions and complications experienced by cutaneous surgeons. *Dermatol Surg.* 2001;27(4):385–390

81. Matzke TJ, Christenson LJ, Christenson SD, et al. Pacemakers and implantable cardiac defibrillators in dermatologic surgery. *Dermatol Surg.* 2006;32(9):1155–1162

82. Koranda FC, Webster RC. Trapdoor effect in nasolabial flaps. Causes and corrections. *Arch Otolaryngol.* 1985;111(7): 421–424

83. Fader DJ, Johnson TM. Ear reconstruction utilizing the subcutaneous island pedicle graft (flip-flop) flap. *Dermatol Surg.* 1999;25(2):94–96

84. Albertini JG. Regarding the modified Burow's wedge flap for upper lateral lip defects. *Dermatol Surg.* 2000;26(10): 981–982

85. Dinehart SM. The rhombic bilobed flap for nasal reconstruction. *Dermatol Surg.* 2001;27(5):501–504

86. Zitelli JA. The bilobed flap for nasal reconstruction. *Arch Dermatol.* 1989;125:957–959

87. Goldminz D, Bennett RG. Cigarette smoking and flap and full-thickness graft necrosis. *Arch Dermatol.* 1991;127: 1012–1015

88. Dixon AJ, Dixon MP. Reducing opposed multilobed flap repair, a new technique for managing medium-sized low-leg defects following skin cancer surgery. *Dermatol Surg.* 2004;30(11):1406–1411

89. Cook JL, Perone JB. A prospective evaluation of the incidence of complications associated with Mohs micrographic surgery. *Arch Dermatol.* 2003;139(2):143–152

90. Amici JM, Rogues AM, Lasheras A, et al. A prospective study of the incidence of complications associated with dermatological surgery. *Br J Dermatol.* 2005;153(5):967–971

91. Colon VF. 10 ways to reduce medical malpractice exposure – doctors, lawyers and lawsuits. Physician Executive March, 2002. At: http://findarticles.com/p/articles/mi_m0843/is_2_28/ai_84236558/pg_1; 2007 Accessed 12.12.07

92. Rice B. 10 ways to guarantee a lawsuit: medical mishaps are only part of the malpractice story. Here's how to prevent the nonclinical errors that get doctors in legal trouble. Medical Economics Jul 8, 2005. At: http://www.memag.com/memag/article/articleDetail.jsp?id=168737&sk=&date=&%0A%09%09%09&pageID=3; 2007 Accessed 12.12.07

Prevention of Keloids

Hillary E. Baldwin

9

9.1 Introduction

Unlike many skin disorders discussed in textbooks, keloids have been described in detail dating back to 3,000 BC.[1] The Yoruba tribe of Western Africa recorded their knowledge of keloids in painting and sculpture ten centuries prior to modern times.[2] Despite this considerable head start, we have made remarkably little progress since the Yorubas toward understanding keloid etiology. This fundamental ignorance is partially responsible for our current lack of consistently reliable, safe treatment, and prevention measures.

Since treatment methods are inadequate in many and challenging in all, prevention becomes vitally important. Here, too, our efforts may be thwarted. There are aspects of keloids that are preventable; one can avoid trauma resulting from voluntary and elective procedures to adorn, augment, or improve. Aggressive prevention of keloids after accidental trauma and necessary surgery is also within our abilities. However, some putative causative factors of keloid formation are out of our control: ethnicity, skin pigmentation, age, gender, and genetic makeup.

This chapter will focus on two aspects of prevention: avoidance techniques for the keloid prone and prevention of recurrence after surgical intervention. First, it will briefly review what is known about keloid epidemiology and pathogenesis to gain insight into the development of a rational prevention plan for these unsightly lesions.

H.E. Baldwin
Department of Dermatology,
SUNY – Brooklyn,
Brooklyn, NY, USA
e-mail: hbaldwin@downstate.edu

9.2 Epidemiology

The reported incidence of keloid formation has ranged from a low of 0.09% in England to a high of 16% in Zaire.[3] Such variation is explained by numerous variables, including race and degree of skin pigmentation. In predominately black and Hispanic populations, incidences between 4.5% and 16% have been reported.[4] Darkly pigmented individuals form keloids 2–19 times more frequently than Caucasians.[5,6] But ethnicity, regardless of pigment intensity, is also a factor. In Aruba, more children of the lighter-skinned Polynesian population form keloids than those of African descent.[7] In Malaysia, those of Chinese decent are more prone to keloid formation than are the darker-skinned Indians and Malays.[8] Although Caucasians form keloids less frequently, those who do can have a very light complexion. These patients are often among the most difficult to treat.

Keloids can occur at any age. New keloid formation is relatively less common in the very young and the elderly. In young children, this may be a function of low trauma frequency and severity. Aging fibroblasts may be less capable of collagen over production.[9,10] Keloid regression after menopause has been reported.[11] In an unpublished study of 212 Caribbean-American and African-American keloid-formers at Kings County Hospital, we found that age as an isolated factor did not correlate with keloid frequency. Rather, the timing of the pierce relative to puberty was predictive of keloid incidence.

Small gender differences that have been reported in the literature are likely to have resulted from cultural trends and reporting bias. Multiple ear pierces are far more common in women than men as are the resulting keloids. Additionally, women may more readily seek medical attention for cosmetic improvement.

R.A. Norman (ed.), *Common Treatments in Preventive Dermatology*,
DOI 10.1007/978-0-85729-853-9_9, © Springer-Verlag London Limited 2012

9.3   Etiology

The plethora of existing theories regarding the etiology of keloids is indicative of our lack of understanding of the condition. The factors that are most consistent are some form of skin trauma occurring in individuals with a genetic predisposition for keloids.

9.3.1   Trauma

"Spontaneous" keloids arising in nontraumatized skin have been suggested. It is more likely however that the severity of the trauma was so minor as to go unnoticed by the patient. Minor abrasions and burns, insect bites, varicella and zoster, vaccinations and tattoos can result in significant keloiding. Acne lesions of the anterior chest and deltoid areas often morph imperceptibly into keloids. Isotretinoin treatment in these patients can prevent additional keloids even when the acne lesions are not readily identifiable. Deep and significant surgical wounds are often less likely to keloid than are the minor wounds described above.

However, trauma is merely the precipitating etiologic factor. Most patients experiencing the same trauma do not keloid. Intrapatient variation is also common. Acne lesions immediately adjacent to each other, bilateral pierces, or adjacent pierces often have different outcomes. Lastly, areas prone to trauma such as the hands and feet rarely keloid.

9.3.2   Skin Tension

Keloids appear most commonly on areas in which skin tension is the highest, namely the anterior chest, upper back, and deltoid areas. The fleshy earlobes are obvious exceptions to this rule. As keloids progress in these areas, they tend to stretch along skin tension lines forming linear or bow-tie shaped lesions.

Closing a wound against the relaxed skin tension lines results in a wound with twice the tension of one closed along Langer's lines.[12] Postsurgical wound tension has been implicated in the literature as a contributing factor in keloid formation.[13,14] The loss of tissue that results from surgical excisions also increases wound tension. Skin grafts may be preferable to primary closure of a tight wound, however, the donor wound may also be subject to keloid formation. The use of tissue expanders to stretch the skin preoperatively offers an alternative that both reduces wound closure tension and applies pressure preoperatively that might help reduce fibroblast function.

Wound tension as a primary etiologic factor in keloid formation loses credibility when one considers the high incidence of earlobe keloids following piercing. The only tension on this wound is that of the minor edema that results from the trauma of the pierce. Chronic edema has been reported to increase glycosaminoglycans (GAGs) in the dermis.[15] It is possible that the chronic edema caused by the pierce (and subsequent reaction to the presence of a metal foreign body) could result in increased incidence of keloid formation.

9.3.3   Infection

There is no evidence to support the supposition that the infectious agents themselves cause keloids. However, the trauma, edema, and increased tension that occur as a result of wound infection might incite keloid formation. This possibility highlights the importance of assiduous avoidance and aggressive treatment of wound infections, especially in the keloid-prone individual.

9.3.4   Endocrine Factors

Multiple and diverse endocrine factors have been associated with keloid incidence although causality is unproven. Keloids have been reported to grow more readily or to appear de novo during pregnancy.[11,13] Keloids have been shown to be more common after puberty than before. This was well known by the Yorubas in the 1600s who knew to pierce ears early in life to prevent keloiding. They also used this knowledge to perfect ritual keloiding in intricate designs after the age of puberty. In our King's County Hospital study, ear pierces that resulted in keloids occurred at a median age of 6.4 years postmenarche, whereas those that did not keloid were pierced at a median age of 4.25 years premenarche.[16]

Melanocyte-stimulating hormone (MSH) has been postulated to play a role in keloid formation. This hypothesis is based on the observation that keloids are more common in patients with hyperpigmentation associated with pregnancy, puberty, and hyperthyroidism. Melanocytes in patients with skin of color may be more reactive to MSH than Caucasians, explaining the higher incidence of keloids in darker-skinned patients. Additionally, keloids are rare on the melanocyte-poor regions of the palms and soles. However, the highly pigmented area of the genitalia is also an infrequent site of keloid formation. Finally, there has never been a reported case of keloid development in an albino patient, even one of African descent.

9.3.5 Genetic Predisposition

Keloids are believed to have a familial predisposition, although the pattern of inheritance is unclear.[3,17] In our study at King's County Hospital, we found a familial pattern in 32% of keloid formers. However, it is possible that the familial tendency to keloid is more a factor of similarity of skin coloration between family members than it is genetically inherited.

9.4 Pathogenesis

Our understanding of keloid pathogenesis is composed of numerous isolated facts that as yet fail to form a cohesive picture. The simple answer to the pathogenesis puzzle is that keloid formation is caused by an increase in anabolic activity in the absence of increased catabolism. Why this happens is not known.

After normal wounding takes place, various signals are sent to the neighboring fibroblasts to increase collagen and GAG production. Upon completion of the rebuilding task, signals are again sent to the fibroblasts to return to their prewound status. Abnormalities in these signals, particularly those that indicate reduction in collagen production, are believed to be responsible for keloid growth. Interferons may be one of those "stop" signals. In normal wounds, there is regression of connective tissue elements after the third week. In keloid tissue, however, fibroblasts proliferate around the plentiful new and dilated capillaries. Collagen

synthesis and GAG synthesis are markedly increased; collagen synthesis is 20 times greater in keloids than in normal skin.[18,19] The absolute number of fibroblasts within the entire keloid is not increased, and they appear histologically normal, but the activity of proline hydroxylase is markedly elevated, suggesting that the rate of collagen biosynthesis is increased in a normally-sized fibroblast population.[18,20] Keloidal fibroblasts also appear to resist programmed cell death.[21,22] Defective apoptosis within keloids may be due to a dysfunctional form of p53. As we will see, injectable interferon may be effective in treating keloids by its enhancement of native p53.

Although collagenase is also increased, collagen degradation is not, possibly due to an increased deposition of alpha-globulins within the keloid.[23,24] Serum alpha-globulins are known inhibitors of collagenase.[23] Estrogens increase the level of serum alpha-globulins, which may help to explain the increased incidence of keloids in pregnant women.[23] Corticosteroids, in contrast, have been shown to reduce the alpha-globulin deposits within keloids.[23] They too may act by increasing activation of collagenase with subsequent breakdown and resorption of the excessive collagen and clinical flattening.

9.5 Preventative Therapy

In any medical inquiry, a literature review of available therapy requires attention to study design and validity of conclusions. This is nowhere more evident than in the field of keloidal scarring in which one must sift through large numbers of anecdotal reports and pure conjecture. The problem begins with the delineation of hypertrophic scars (HTSs) from keloids. Many studies include both entities in the admittance criteria yet fail to reveal, which lesions ultimately responded to therapy. Other patient and lesion characteristics routinely omitted from these studies include such important factors as patient race and age, lesion age and symptomatology, lesion size and location, recurrence vs. virgin lesion and lesion morphology (sessile vs. pedunculated or dome-shaped). Most reports also suffer from inadequate follow-up time of less than 6 months. It is an undisputable truth that keloid removal is easy; the trick is preventing recurrence or occurrence.

In a recent review article, Shaffer et al. conclude that despite a plethora of papers on the topic of keloids, "there are no definitive treatment protocols."[25] This is a result of poorly designed and uncontrolled studies in which the endpoint of therapy (cosmesis, function, or symptoms) is rarely identified. Only radiation therapy (RT) in combination with surgery met their standards for proven therapy. Mustoe et al. also lamented the absence of well-controlled studies and concluded that corticosteroid injection and silicone gel sheeting (SGS) are the "… only treatments for which sufficient evidence exists to make evidence-based recommendations."[26] Durani and Bayat found SGS and laser therapy to have the highest level of support, albeit subpar.[27] Leventhal et al. noted that "most treatments for keloidal and hypertrophic scarring offer minimal likelihood of improvement."[28] Other treatments at this time are still lacking the proof of efficacy that arises only from a well-designed, randomized, placebo-controlled trial with adequate patient numbers. The nature of keloid therapy is such that a comparison of various techniques is often not amenable to double-blinding. We look forward to more studies in which single techniques are compared to controls, vehicles, or dummy therapy.

At the present time, we must recognize that keloid prevention techniques are not necessarily evidence-based. We are using techniques for which definitive data does not exist. Presented below are the techniques that have become the standard of care in the field.

9.5.1 Corticosteroids

Because of their ease of administration, low cost, and low risk, intralesional corticosteroids alone and in combination are the work horses of keloid occurrence and recurrence prevention. Although no solid evidence-based literature supports their use in this role, they have become the first-line approach of most physicians dealing with this condition worldwide.

9.5.1.1 Corticosteroids as Monotherapy for Keloid Prevention

Triamcinolone acetonide (TAC) is the most commonly utilized corticosteroid. Concentrations from 10 to 40 mg/kg are used. Injections can be repeated every 2–4 weeks, depending on the total dose of steroid used and the size of the injected space. The most common cause of steroid "failure" is the use of inadequate concentrations. Concentrations less than 10 mg/mL are rarely effective in prevention. To avoid the risk of hypothalamic-pituitary axis suppression, this author does not inject more than 40 mg/session. This means that the total area treated in one session will be limited by total safe dose constraints. Better to inject an efficacious dose in a smaller area than to spread it so thin that it is ineffective. This concept must be kept in mind when planning the surgical excision of an existing keloid. It is imprudent to remove more keloid volume than can be subsequently injected for recurrence prevention; staged excisions may therefore be preferable. Although additional areas may be injected on the following weeks, it is best not to inject the same area with high doses at less than 2-week intervals. The depot effect of the injected steroids is such that repeat injections done too frequently can result in atrophy. Hypopigmentation is also more likely in this setting. With subsequent treatments, the strength of the steroid is often reduced in order to fine-tune the ultimate outcome.

9.5.1.2 Corticosteroids as Part of Polytherapy for Keloid Prevention

Corticosteroids can be combined with any other treatment modality to improve outcome. Following surgical excision, many authors have shown a reduction in recurrence rates with the addition of postoperative corticosteroids.[29,30] Combinations with cryotherapy and silicone gel sheets have been shown to be superior to either modality alone.[31] Corticosteroids plus alpha interferon have been shown to be more effective than corticosteroids alone.[32,33] Combinations with lasers and alpha interferon also have shown promise (see Sect. 9.5.10).[34]

Corticosteroids are an integral part of keloid prevention – both de novo occurrence in a new surgical wound and recurrence following keloid excision. This author follows the following injection schedule. On the day of surgery, and then at 2, 4, and 6 weeks, the wound margins are injected with TAC 40 mg/mL regardless of the appearance of the wound. At 2 months, and every month thereafter, injections are given as clinically necessary. At that point, dosage of the corticosteroids given at each session is determined clinically by the site, size, degree of firmness, and symptoms the patient is experiencing. Preventative therapy is best carried out for 1 full year; early discontinuation is associated with a higher incidence of unnecessary recurrences.

Common side effects of steroid injections include hypopigmentation and skin atrophy. The hypopigmentation can be pronounced and may last 6–12 months before resolving. However, hypopigmentation can also be used as a marker of clinical success. Both hypopigmentation and atrophy can be reduced by avoiding injecting into the surrounding normal tissue. Skin atrophy is often a necessary consequence of adequate therapy. After treatment, the atrophic surface may appear wrinkled or shiny, and telangiectasias are common. This appearance improves with time. Alternatively, vascular lasers can be utilized to lessen the telangiectasias.

9.5.2 Surgical Methods to Prevent Keloid Recurrence

Surgical removal of large, bulky keloids is often necessary. However, monotherapy results in a high incidence of recurrence, often 50–100%.[30,35] Surgery must be combined with adjunctive techniques such as RT, steroids, or interferon.

9.5.2.1 Use the Smallest Incision as Possible

The smallest incision possible is made, extending less than the entire length of the keloid. Dissect off any usable epidermis from the keloid for ease of closure.

9.5.2.2 Remove all Keloidal Tissue

Unless it would result in gross deformity or loss of function, all of the keloid material should be removed. Care should be taken to remove any trapped hairs.

9.5.2.3 Minimize Wound Tension

Closure should be done with the least amount of tension. Surgery followed by grafting alone results in a superior nonrecurrence rate over primary closure

(59%).[17] However, donor-site keloids are likely. As a result, tissue expanders may be preferable.

9.5.2.4 Suture Considerations

Whenever possible monofilament suture should be used to reduce the incidence of wound infection, abscess formation and inflammation along the suture line. Sutures often need to be left in longer than usual to prevent dehiscence. This is especially true when steroids are injected postoperatively. If the resulting wound is fairly superficial or very broad, and the patient is amenable, allowing the wound to heal by secondary intention often results in better cosmetic outcome and a lower incidence of recurrence.

9.5.3 Earlobe Keloids

Earlobes keloids need to be considered separately. Many authors have noted a lower rate of keloid recurrence in the earlobe.[36,37] Studies have shown a recurrence rate of only 41% respectively after surgery alone.[38] Studies utilizing both surgery and steroids have shown recurrence rates of 1–20%.[39-41] Surgery with adjunctive RT has resulted in recurrence rates of 0–8.6%.[39,42-44] With careful, aggressive therapy and using multiple modalities, earlobe keloids rarely recur.

Better surgical results on earlobes are probably the result of several factors. First-time earlobe lesions tend to be very discrete, and easily separated from the surrounding dermis and epidermis. Complete removal of all keloidal tissue is thus easier to accomplish. Most earlobe keloids occur in women who are profoundly motivated to wear earrings again, and are far more compliant than the average keloid patient. The fleshy tissue of the ear makes closure without tension easier to accomplish. Postoperative pressure is easily applied with the use of pressure earrings. These earrings are not particularly cosmetically appealing, but the patients find them easy to wear and comfortable. They also make an ideal postoperative dressing, obviating the need for bulky, and often, inadequate pressure dressings.

9.5.4 Laser Surgery

After initial excitement over the demonstrated ability of the CO_2 laser to decrease fibroblast activity in vitro, its use in keloid therapy was a disappointment.[44-47] Used in the defocused mode, recurrence rate is extremely high.[48] In the focused mode, recurrence rate is similar to surgery alone (50–70%).[46,49] The Nd-YAG laser has been demonstrated to cause an in vitro selective bioinhibition of collagen production, but recurrence rates of 53–100% in vivo.[50] The pulsed dye laser (PDL) has been reported to improve hypertrophic scar (HTS) symptoms, decrease scar height, and improve skin texture. Alster and Williams showed a 57–83% improvement with the 585 nm flashpump PDL in the prevention of keloids in sternotomy scars.[51] They noted the importance of starting therapy early for the best results. It has been proposed that the PDL decreases the microvasculature in early keloids and HTSs resulting in anoxia. Several combination studies have shown that PDL works better in combination with other modalities, including corticosteroids, interferon, and carbon dioxide laser.[24,52-55]

9.5.5 Radiation Therapy

The mechanism of action of RT in prevention of keloids is unknown. It may decrease fibroblast collagen synthesis.[56] Alternatively, it may act by decreasing vascular hyperplasia.[57]

For prophylaxis in keloid-prone individuals, X-radiation, electron beam, and interstitial radiation have all been reported to result in similar cure rates (recurrence rates near 20%, which are far superior to other modalities).[58-60] Dosing schedule and fractionation have varied greatly from one study to another, but outcomes are similar. A minimum of 1,000 rad or equivalent appears to be the common consensus for successful outcome.[61] Kal and Veen concluded that RT should be done within 2 days of surgical removal, and that short treatment durations and "relatively high doses" are necessary.[62] In a study of earlobe keloids, surgery plus RT was compared to surgery plus corticosteroids.[39] Recurrence rates were 12.5 and of 33%, respectively. Recurrence rates of 4.7% with high-dose-rate brachytherapy,[63] 21% with interstitial iridium-192,[64] 16, 19, and 32% with electron beam[65-67] have been demonstrated.

Recurrence rates have been shown to be higher in areas of high tension such as the chest, scapula, and suprapubic areas in three studies.[66-68] The short treatment plan required with RT may aid in patient compliance.

Despite its high incidence of success in preventing keloid recurrence, RT is avoided by many clinicians due to largely unfounded concerns regarding the long-term risks of malignancy of the skin or underlying structures. Numerous large studies report a 0% carcinogenesis rate.[61] Only one reported case of squamous cell carcinoma arising in postkeloid radiation site is evident in the literature, and the causality is unclear.[69] Botwood et al. attempted to put these concerns into perspective.[61] In more than 100 years in clinical use, there are only three case reports of malignancies occurring postkeloid RT. Breast cancer in a 57-year-old woman occurring 29 years after RT to a chest keloid was reported in 1999.[61] Breast cancer in a 36-year-old woman 23 years after chest wall keloid radiation was reported in 1982[70] In both cases, confounding variables were also evident (7-year history of hormone replacement therapy and evidence of unusually high radiation doses, respectively). A single case report of thyroid cancer occurring in a 27-year-old man 8 years after RT to a keloid of the chin has also been reported.[71] Histopathology revealed a *medullary* carcinoma; radiation-induced carcinomas of the thyroid are exclusively *papillary* carcinomas.[72] Based on dosimetry studies, RT in standard dosages to the ear with proper shielding would expose the ipsilateral thyroid lobe to only two rads.[61] Studies therefore do not warrant a high level of concern. Common side effects to consider are skin atrophy, radiation dermatitis, abnormal skin pigmentation, and local alopecia. RT is not recommended in children with keloids; if used, metaphyses must be shielded to prevent retardation of bone growth, which may occur at doses of 400 R and less.[73]

9.5.6 Compression Therapy

Compression therapy – applying pressure greater than that of capillary pressure (24 mmHg) – causes a reduction in soft tissue cellularity. Histopathology shows increased interstitial space and collagen bundles that are more widely dispersed.[74] It is theorized that pressure creates hypoxia resulting in fibroblast degeneration and subsequent collagen degradation.

Dressings, which apply 15–45 mmHg, worn 24 h a day for 4–6 months are often successful in reducing keloid recurrence rates postoperatively. Not all areas are amenable to pressure dressings, which in any event are uncomfortable, hot, and unsightly. Ears are the exception to this rule. Newer pressure earrings have large compression plates that are more comfortable to wear. "Sleeper" styles are less bulky and less conspicuous.

9.5.7 Silicone Products

SGS has been touted in many studies to be efficacious in preventing the development of HTSs and keloids.[75-77] These studies are marred by the absence of blinding and control, small patient numbers and inadequate follow-up time. SGS has been shown in small studies to reduce HTS formation by as much as 70% when used consistently.[77] It must be worn over a scar for 2–3 months, 12–24 h a day to prevent development.[78] Sheets are available in varying thicknesses and consistency. Adhesive tape is necessary for consistent application. A new formulation of silicone gel has recently been reported.[79,80] The gel is self-drying and forms a flexible and transparent sheet after application, obviating the need for tape.

The mechanism of action of SGS is unknown. SGS is known to retard epidermal water loss. The drier agents have been shown to create static electricity, which some believe to play a role in its effectiveness. In a controlled, prospective nonblinded study, SGS was compared to an occlusive dressing without silicone.[81] SGS was not found to be superior, leading the authors to conclude that it was wound hydration, not the presence of silicone that was responsible for the clinical effect.

9.5.8 Interferon

As discussed previously, fibroblast activity increases dramatically after wounding. Once the wound is adequately stabilized, signals are sent to the fibroblasts to shut off this excessive production of ground substance and collagen. Interferons are one of these signals. Berman and Duncan reported that short-term intralesional interferon

alpha-2b treatment of a keloid resulted in a selective and persistent normalization of keloidal fibroblast collagen, GAG and collagenase production in vitro, and a rapid reduction in the area of the keloid.[82] Interferon has also been shown to upregulate native p53 that is dysfunctional in keloidal fibroblasts.[83] This might promote the natural cell death of the over-active fibroblasts.

Both alpha and gamma interferon are available for use. Initial clinical trials with gamma interferon were disappointing and it is no longer in use.[84] Granstein has reported on an unpublished study where 18 of 19 keloid reexcisions were accomplished without recurrence at 1 year by two postoperative injections of interferon alpha (Granstein, Personal communication, 1996). Berman reported response in 11/12 recurrent keloids of the head and neck after surgical excision and interferon alpha 2b.[85] Berman and Flores reported a recurrence rate of 51.5% following surgery alone, 58.4% after surgery and corticosteroids, and 18.7% when surgery was combined with both interferon and corticosteroid injections.[32] At Kings County Hospital, we have found that interferon alpha injections can be used to decrease keloid recurrence after earlobe keloid excisions in which keloidal tissue was left behind.

Injections of interferon alpha-2b are done on the day of surgery and then 1 week postoperatively directly into the wound. One million units per linear centimeter are injected into the wound base and margins. In the case of a wound allowed to heal by secondary intention, injections are given approximately every square centimeter. Side effects are reduced by limiting total dose to less than five million units per treatment.

Side effects of interferon alpha-2b include a flu-like syndrome, which can be reduced or eliminated by the prophylactic use of acetaminophen, and timing of the injection late in the afternoon so that mild febrile reactions pass unnoticed during sleep.

9.5.9 Imiquimod Application

Imiquimod 5% cream is a potent and rapid inducer of interferon after topical application. Topical application of imiquimod to keloids has been shown to significantly alter gene expression of markers of apoptosis.[83] As such, its use in keloid therapy was a logical continuance from injectable interferon. Berman and Kaufman reported its use postoperatively in an uncontrolled pilot study of 13 keloids removed from 12 patients.[86] Applications were done twice daily, beginning on the day of surgery and continuing for 8 weeks. At 24 weeks, none of 11 keloids (ten earlobe, one trunk) evaluated had recurred. The authors have subsequently reported one recurrence in the lesion removed from the back.

Since then, several other small, uncontrolled trials have suggested that imiquimod is most effective on the earlobes. Stashower showed no recurrence at 12 months in four patients with eight earlobe keloids.[87] Martin-Garcia and Busquets reported a 25% recurrence rate in eight earlobe keloids.[88] Chaungsuwanich and Gunjittisomram showed an overall 6-month recurrence rate of 28.6% in 35 patients.[89] Recurrences on the pinna were rare (2.9%) and those of the chest common (83.3%). Malhotra et al. showed an improvement after surgical excision of three presternal keloids in two patients over the 8-week treatment phase, but recurrence 4 weeks later in all patients.[90] In an ongoing study, we have found a modest reduction in keloid recurrence in nonearlobe keloids treated with imiquimod. In a placebo-controlled, double-blind study of six patients with 12 nonadjacent keloids, we found a 50% reduction in keloid reformation. The recurrences in the imiquimod-treated areas occurred later and were easier to treat than placebo-treated recurrences. More controlled studies need to be performed to assess the effectiveness of this treatment modality.

In all of the studies mentioned, there were few topical and no systemic side effects noted. Application of imiquimod to open wounds was mostly nonirritating. Discontinuation for several days was adequate to control this unlikely side effect.

9.5.10 Combination Therapy

There is no medical reason to limit preventative treatment to a single agent or modality. Prevention of recurrence or occurrence can be greatly improved when all available modalities are utilized simultaneously. Interferon injections at day 1 and day 8 combined with RT can deliver two adjunctive therapies in the first 2 weeks post-op when patient compliance is at its peak. Pressure dressings if possible, imiquimod application

and continue corticosteroid injections as previously delineated can be used in conjunction to maximize outcome.

9.6 Keloid Avoidance Behaviors

The first goal of therapy is, of course, prevention of unnecessary trauma. Cosmetic procedures should be discouraged. Ears from which keloids have been removed should not be repierced.

Early and aggressive treatment of accidental wounds or nonelective surgeries is crucial in keloid-prone individuals. Necessary surgical procedures should be closed parallel to relaxed skin tension lines with minimal stress. Skin grafts, tissue expanders, and healing by secondary intention should be considered to minimize wound tension. Wounds should be covered with SGS and/or pressure garments whenever possible. Preventative intralesional corticosteroids should be injected at the time of the procedure and regularly thereafter. Intralesional interferon and RT should also be considered. Often this must be coordinated in advance with the patient's general surgeon. Such interference is not always appreciated and it is prudent to elicit the help of the patient in convincing the surgeon of the importance of early intervention.

Patients in whom acne lesions tend to form keloids must be carefully monitored and treated. They should be educated to present at the first sign of an inflammatory acne lesion for intralesional steroids. Multiple lesions are an indication for oral antibiotics or a course of isotretinoin. Similarly, in dark-skinned individuals with a family history of keloid formation, varicella or zoster should be aggressively treated with antiviral agents.

9.7 Summary

Keloids are a challenging problem for which there is no quick fix, or indeed the promise of a fix at all. Beyond the futility of telling a patient not to get injured, many aspects of keloids cannot be changed. Age, ethnicity, skin coloration, genetic makeup, and hormonal influences are not alterable. Preventative care therefore, is more focused on prevention of occurrence of new lesions in a keloid-prone individual and the prevention of recurrence after surgical removal.

References

1. Breasted JH. *The Edwin Smith Surgical Papyrus, Vol I: Hieroglyphic Translation and Commentary.* Chicago: University of Chicago; 1930:403–406
2. Omo-Dare P. Yoruban contribution to literature on keloids. *J Nat Med Assoc.* 1973;65:367–406
3. Bloom D. Heredity of keloids: review of the literature and report of a family with multiple keloids for five generations. *N Y State J Med.* 1956;56:511
4. Abrahms B, Benedetto A, Humeniuk H. Exuberant keloidal formation. *JAOAC Int.* 1993;93:863–865
5. Brenizer A. Keloid formation in the Negro. *Ann Surg.* 1915; 61:87
6. Fox H. Observations on skin diseases in the American Negro. *J Cutan Dis.* 1908;26:67
7. Alhady SM, Sivanantharajah K. Keloids in various races; a review of 175 cases. *Plast Reconstr Surg.* 1969;44:564
8. Arnold H, Graver F. Keloids: etiology and management. *Arch Dermatol.* 1959;80:772
9. Rockwell W, Cohen I, Ehrlich H. Keloids and hypertrophic scars. A comprehensive review. *Plast Reconstr Surg.* 1989; 84:827–837
10. Davies D. Scars, hypertrophic scars and keloids. *Plast Reconstr Surg.* 1985;290:1056–1058
11. Kelly P. Keloids. *Dermatol Clin.* 1988;6:413–424
12. Flint M. The biological basis of Langer's lines. In: Longacre JJ, ed. *The Ultrastructure of Collagen.* Springfield IL: Charles C Thomas; 1976:132–140
13. Stucker F, Shaw G. An approach to management of keloids. *Arch Otolaryngol Head Neck Surg.* 1992;118:63–67
14. Asboe-Hansen G. Hypertrophic scars and keloids; etiology, pathogenesis and dermatologic therapy. *Dermatologia.* 1960;120:178
15. Kormoczy B. Enormous keloid (?) on a penis. *Br J Plast Surg.* 1978;31:268
16. Lane J, Waller J, Davis L. Relationship between age of ear piercing and keloid formation. *Pediatrics.* 2005;115: 1312–1314
17. Cosman B, Crikelair G, Ju M, Gaulin J, Lattes R. The surgical treatment of keloids. *Plast Reconstr Surg.* 1961; 27:335–345
18. Abergel R, Pizzurro D, Meeker C, et al Biochemical composition of the connective tissue in keloids and analysis of collagen metabolism in keloid fibroblast cultures. *J Invest Dermatol.* 1985;84:384–390
19. Cohen I, Keiser H, Sjoerdsma A. Collagen synthesis in human keloid patients. *Plast Reconstr Surg.* 1979;63:689
20. Tan E, Rouda S, Greenbaum S, et al Acidic and basic fibroblast growth factors downregulate collagen gene expression in keloid fibroblasts. *Am J Pathol.* 1993;142:463–470
21. Sayah DN, Soo C, Shaw WW, et al Downregulation of apoptosis-related genes in keloid tissues. *J Surg Res.* 1999;87: 209–216
22. Akasaka Y, Fujita K, Ishikawa Y, et al Detection of apoptosis in keloids and a comparative study on apoptosis between keloids, hypertrophic scars, normal healed fibrotic scars, and dermatofibroma. *Wound Repair Regen.* 2001;9:501–506
23. Diegelmann R, Bryant C, Cohen I. Tissue alpha globulins in keloid formation. *Plast Reconstr Surg.* 1977;59:481
24. Bauer E, Eisen A, Jeffrey J. Regulation of vertebrate collagenase activity in vivo and in vitro. *J Invest Dermatol.* 1972;59:50–55
25. Shaffer J, Taylor S, Cook-Bolden F. Keloidal scars: a review with a critical look at therapeutic options. *J Am Acad Dermatol.* 2002;46:S63–S97
26. Mustoe T, Cooter R, Gold M, et al International clinical recommendations on scar management. *Plast Reconstr Surg.* 2002;110:560–571
27. Durani P, Bayat A. Levels of evidence for the treatment of keloid disease. *J Plast Reconstr Aesthet Surg.* 2008;61:4–17
28. Lenventhal D, Furr M, Reiter D. Treatment of keloids and hypertrophic scars: a meta-analysis and review of the literature. *Arch Facial Plast Surg.* 2006;8:362–368
29. Lahiri A, Tsilihoti D, Gaze N. Experience with difficult keloids. *Br J Plast Surg.* 2001;54:633–635
30. Lawrence W. In search of the optimal treatment of keloids: report of a series and a review of the literature. *Ann Plast Surg.* 1991;27:164–178
31. Yosipovitch G, Widijanti Sugene M, Goon A, et al A Comparison of the combined effect of cryotherapy and corticosteroid injections versus corticosteroids and cryotherapy on keloids: a controlled study. *J Dermatol Treat.* 2001;12:87–90
32. Berman B, Flores F. Recurrence rates of excised keloids treated with postoperative triamcinolone injections of interferon alpha 2b. *J Am Acad Dermatol.* 1997;37:755–757
33. Lee J, Kim S, Lee A. Effects of interferon-alpha2b on keloid treatment with triamcinolone acetonide intralesional injection. *Int J Dermatol.* 2008;47:183–186
34. Akoz T, Gideroglu K, Akan M. Combination of different techniques for the treatment of earlobe keloids. *Aesthetic Plast Surg.* 2002;26:184–188
35. Darzi M, Chowdi N, Kaul S, et al Evaluation of various methods of treating keloids and hypertrophic scars: a 10-year follow-up study. *Br J Plast Surg.* 1992;45:374–379
36. Ogawa R, Miyashita T, Hyakusoku H, et al Postoperative radiation protocol for keloids and hypertrophic scars: statistical analysis of 370 sites followed for over 18 months. *Ann Plast Surg.* 2007;59:688–691
37. Narkwong L, Thirakhupt P. Postoperative radiotherapy with high-dose-rate iridium 192 mould for prevention of earlobe keloids. *J Med Assoc Thai.* 2006;89:428–433
38. Rauscher G, Kolmer W. Treatment of recurrent earlobe keloids. *Cutis.* 1996;38:67–68

39. Sclafani A, Gordon L, Chadha M, Romo T. Prevention of earlobe keloid recurrence with postoperative corticosteroid injections versus radiation therapy. *Dermatol Surg*. 1996;22: 569–574

40. Shons A, Press B. The treatment of earlobe keloids by surgical excision and postoperative triamcinolone injection. *Ann Plast Surg*. 1983;10:480–482

41. Rosen D, Patel M, Freeman K, Weiss P. A primary protocol for the management of ear keloids: results of excision combined with intraoperative and postoperative steroid injections. *Plast Reconstr Surg*. 2007;120:1395–1400

42. Akita S, Akino K, Yakabe A, et al Combined surgical excision and radiation therapy for keloid treatment. *J Craniofac Surg*. 2007;18:1164–1169

43. Ragoowansi R, Cornes P, Glees J, et al Earlobe keloids: treatment by a protocol of surgical excision and immediate postoperative adjuvant radiotherapy. *Br J Plast Surg*. 2001;54: 504–508

44. Chaudhry M, Akhtar S, Duvalsaint F, et al Earlobe keloids, surgical excision followed by radiation therapy: a 10-year experience. *Ear Nose Throat J*. 1994;73:779–781

45. Stern J, Lucente F. Carbon dioxide laser excision of earlobe keloids. *Arch Otolaryngol Head Neck Surg*. 1988;113: 1107–1111

46. Kantor G, Wheeland R, Bailin P, et al Treatment of earlobe keloids with carbon dioxide laser excision: a report of 16 cases. *J Dermatol Surg Oncol*. 1985;11:1063–1067

47. Driscoll B. Treating keloids with carbon dioxide lasers. *Arch Otolaryngol Head Neck Surg*. 2001;127:1145

48. Alster T. Laser treatment of hypertrophic scars, keloids, and striae. *Dermatol Clin*. 1997;15:419–429

49. Apfelberg D, Maser M, White D, Lash H. Failure of carbon dioxide laser excision of keloids. *Lasers Surg Med*. 1989;9: 382–388

50. Sherman R, Rosenfeld H. Experience with the NDYAG laser in the treatment of keloid scars. *Ann Plast Surg*. 1988;24: 231–233

51. Alster T, Williams C. Treatment of keloid sternotomy scars with 585 nm flashlamp-pumped pulsed-dye laser. *Lancet*. 1995;345:118–200

52. Connell P, Harland C. Treatment of keloid scars with pulsed dye laser and intralesional steroids. *J Cutan Laser Ther*. 2000;2:147–159

53. Maniskiatti W, Fitzpatrick R. Treatment response of keloidal and hypertrophic, sternotomy scars: comparison among intralesional corticosteroid, 5-fluorouracil, and 585-nm flash-lamp-pumped pulsed-dye laser treatments. *Arch Dermatol*. 2002;138:1149–1155

54. Asilian A, Darougheh A, Shariati F. New combination of triamcinolone, 5-fluorouracil, and pulsed-dye laser for treatment of keloid and hypertrophic scars. *Dermatol Surg*. 2006;32:907–915

55. Alster T, Handrick C. Laser treatment of hypertrophic scars, keloids, and striae. *Semin Cutan Med Surg*. 2000;19:287–292

56. Order S, Donaldsen S. *Radiation Therapy for Benign Disease*. Springer; 1990:147–153

57. Borok T, Brav M, Sinclair I, et al Role of ionizing irradiation for 393 keloids. *Int J Radiat Oncol Biol Phys*. 1988;15:865–870

58. Ollstein R, Siegel H, Gillooley J, et al Treatment of keloids by combined surgical excision and immediate postoperative X-ray therapy. *Ann Plast Surg*. 1981;7:281–285

59. Khumpar D, Murray J, Anscher M. Keloids treated with excision followed by radiation therapy. *J Am Acad Dermatol*. 1994;31:225–231

60. Darzi M, Chowdi N, Kaul S, Kahn M. Evaluation of various methods of treating keloids and hypertrophic scars: a 10-year experience. *Int J Radiat Oncol Biol Phys*. 1989;17:77–80

61. Botwood N, Lewanski C, Lowdell C. The risks of treating keloids with radiotherapy. *Br J Radiol*. 1999;72:1222–1224

62. Kal H, Veen R. Biologically effective doses of postoperative radiotherapy in the prevention of keloids. Dose-effect relationship. *Strahlenther Onkol*. 2005;181:717–723

63. Guix B, Henriquez I, Andres A, et al Treatment of keloids by high-dose-rate brachytherapy. *Int J Radiat Oncol Biol Phys*. 2001;50:167–172

64. Escarmant P, Zimmerman S, Amar A, et al The treatment of 783 keloid scars by iridium 192 interstitial radiation after surgical excision. *Int J Radiat Oncol Biol Phys*. 1993;26:245–251

65. Maarouf M, Schleicher U, Schmachtenberg A, Ammon J. Radiotherapy in the management of keloids. Clinical experience with electron beam irradiation and comparison with X-ray therapy. *Strahlenther Onkol*. 2002;178:330–335

66. Bischof M, Krempien R, Debus J, Treiber M. Postoperative electron beam radiotherapy for keloids: objective findings and patient satisfaction in self-assessment. *Int J Dermatol*. 2007;46:971–975

67. Ogawa R, Mitsuhashi K, Hyakusoku H, Miyashita T. Postoperative electron-beam irradiation therapy for keloids and hypertrophic scars: retrospective study of 147 cases followed for more than 18 months. *Plast Reconstr Surg*. 2003;111:547–553

68. Wagner W, Alfrink M, Micke O, et al Results of prophylactic irradiation in patients with resected keloids: a retrospective analysis. *Acta Oncol*. 2000;39:217–220

69. Mizuno H, Cagri Uysal A, Koike S, Hyakusoku H. Squamous cell carcinoma of the auricle arising from keloid after radium needle therapy. *J Craniofac Surg*. 2006;17:360–362

70. Bilbey J, Muller N, Miller R, Nelemus B. Localized fibrous mesothelioma of pleura following external ionizing radiation therapy. *Chest*. 1988;94:1291–1292

71. Hoffman S. Radiotherapy for keloids? *Ann Plast Surg*. 1982; 9:265

72. Sampson R, Kev C, Buschler C, Iijima S. Thyroid carcinoma and radiation. *JAMA*. 1969;209:65

73. Doornbos J, Stoffel T, Hass A, et al The role of kilovoltage irradiation in the treatment of keloids. *Int J Radiat Oncol Biol Phys*. 1990;18:833–838

74. Kosaka M, Kamiishi H. New concept of balloon-compression wear for the treatment of keloids and hypertrophic scars. *Plast Reconstr Surg*. 2001;108:1454–1455

75. Gold M. A controlled clinical trial of topical silicone gel sheeting in the treatment of hypertrophic scars and keloids. *J Am Acad Dermatol*. 1994;30:506–507

76. Fulton J. Silicone gel sheeting for the prevention and management of evolving hypertrophic and keloid scars. *Dermatol Surg*. 1995;21:947–951

77. Ahn S, Monafo W, Mustoe T. Topical silicone gel: a new treatment for hypertrophic scars. *Surgery*. 1989;106:781–786

78. Berman B, Perez O, Konda S, et al A review of the biologic effects, clinical efficacy, and safety of silicone elastomer sheeting for hypertrophic and keloid scar treatment and management. *Dermatol Surg*. 2007;33:1291–1302

79. Mustoe T. Evolution of silicone therapy and mechanism of action in scar management. *Aesthetic Plast Surg*. 2008;32: 82–92

80. Signorini M, Clementoni M. Clinical evaluation of a new self-drying silicone gel in the treatment of scars: a preliminary report. *Aesthetic Plast Surg*. 2007;31(2):183–187

81. Viana de Oliveira G, Nunes T, Magna L, et al Silicone versus nonsilicone gel dressings: a controlled trial. *Dermatol Surg*. 2001;27:721–726

82. Berman N, Duncan M. Short-term keloid treatment in vivo with human interferon alfa-2b results in a selective and persistent normalization of keloidal fibroblast collagen, glycosaminoglycans and collagenase production in vitro. *J Am Acad Dermatol*. 1989;21(4 Pt 1):694–702

83. Jacob S, Berman B, Vincek V. Topical application of imiquimod 5% cream to keloids alters expression genes associated with apoptosis. *Br J Dermatol*. 2008;149:62–65

84. Granstein R, Rook A, Flotte T, et al Intralesional interferon gamma treatment for keloids and hypertrophic scars. *Arch Otolaryngol Head Neck Surg*. 1990;118:1159–1162

85. Berman B, Bieley H. Adjunct therapies of surgical management of keloids. *Dermatol Surg*. 1996;22:126–130

86. Berman B, Kaufman J. Pilot study of the effect of postoperative imiquimod 5% cream recurrence rate of excised keloids. *J Am Acad Dermatol*. 2002;47:S209–S211

87. Stashower M. Successful treatment of earlobe keloids with imiquimod after tangential shave excision. *Dermatol Surg*. 2006;32:380–386

88. Martin-Garcia R, Busquets A. Postsurgical use of imiquimod 5% cream in the prevention of earlobe keloid recurrences: results of an open-label, pilot study. *Dermatol Surg*. 2005;31:1394–1398

89. Chuangsuwanich A, Gunjittisomram S. The efficacy of 5% imiquimod cream in the prevention of recurrence of excised keloids. *J Med Assoc Thai*. 2007;90:1363–1367

90. Malhotra A, Gupta S, Khaitan B, Sharma V. Imiquimod 5% cream for the prevention of recurrence after excision of presternal keloids. *Dermatology*. 2007;215:63–65

Index

R.A. Norman (ed.), *Common Treatments in Preventive Dermatology,*
DOI 10.1007/978-0-85729-853-9, © Springer-Verlag London Limited 2012